# A MINUTE FOR
# YOUR HEALTH

# A MINUTE FOR YOUR HEALTH

⸺⟨∿⟩⸺

## THE ABC'S FOR IMPROVED HEALTH AND LONGEVITY

*Edited for*

*The Association of Black Cardiologists*

*by*

*Stephanie H. Kong, M.D.*

HILTON PUBLISHING COMPANY • ROSCOE, ILLINOIS

ISBN 0–9675258–9–6

Hilton Publishing Company
PO Box 737, Roscoe, IL 61073
815-885-1070
www.hiltonpub.com

To obtain additional copies or information about this book contact:

Association of Black Cardiologists, Inc.
6849 B2 Peachtree-Dunwoody Road
Atlanta, GA 30328
800/753–9222
678/302–4222

You may also visit our website: www.abcardio.org

# CONTENTS

vii

# ABOUT THE EDITOR AND THE ASSOCIATION OF BLACK CARDIOLOGISTS, INC.

## Stephanie H. Kong, M.D.

In addition to the clinical practice of medicine, Dr. Stephanie Kong has dedicated her career to improving the health of African Americans by developing strategies to empower adults to take control of their health and motivate others to do likewise. As a Pediatric Resident at Milwaukee Children's Hospital, she authored a practical guide for mothers, *Hey Mom, Did you Know?*, which emphasized active participation of mothers in the health of their children. Dr. Kong has spent most of her professional career as a managed care executive. She has served on the clinical faculty of the Medical College of Wisconsin, Penn State- Hershey Medical Center and Johns Hopkins University School of Medicine. She has authored several publications on managed care, quality of life and preventive medicine. She is currently the Chair of the Cultural Competence Committee of the Association of Black Cardiologists and resides in Atlanta.

### The Association of Black Cardiologists, Inc.
The ABC was founded by 17 progressive cardiologists and scientists at the American Heart Association annual meeting in Dallas, TX in 1974. They dedicated the organization to reducing the cardiovascular disease burden in the African American community.

The original intent was to partner with government, industry, foundations, churches and professional organizations, as well as to make membership available to all who are concerned about the reduced life expectancy of African Americans.

The American Heart Association provided staff support (Mr. Glen Bennett), and Dr. Richard Allen Williams, our founder, served as President for the first twelve years. In 1986, the by-laws were changed, Dr. B. Waine Kong was hired as the Chief Executive Officer and a succession of incredibly innovative presidents (Drs. Daniel Savage, Elijah Saunders, Jay Brown, Augustus Grant, Paul Douglass, Frank James, Elizabeth Ofili and Malcolm Taylor) contributed to the success of the organization and the reduction of heart disease and stroke in our community.

With the recognition that by age 21, due to cardiovascular disease, African American children are fortunate if they have even one surviving grandparent, in 1997, the ABC adopted the mantra "Children Should Know Their Grandparents and become GREAT Grandparents Themselves". This slogan has galvanized the community and solidified our commitment to reducing our susceptibility to cardiovascular disease. If we want to meet those wonderful people in our future, we must take better care of ourselves today.

In order to improve the quality of life and longevity for African Americans, the ABC promotes:

1. The development of culturally competent health care providers.
2. Equal access to medical care and innovative technologies.
3. Greater access to African American physicians, specialists and other health professionals.
4. Preventive, holistic health with our recommended Seven Steps to Good Health for African Americans.

# FOREWORD

## By Dale A. Matthews, MD, FACP

*Associate Professor of Medicine,*
*Georgetown University School of Medicine, Washington, D.C.*
Author, The Faith Factor: Proof of the Healing Power of
Prayer *(N.Y., Viking, 1998)*

*The fear of the LORD is the beginning of wisdom and knowledge of*
*the Holy One is understanding. For through me your days will be*
*many and years will be added to your life.*
ઓ Proverbs 9:10–11, NIV

Since the days of Solomon, the wise have recognized that religious commitment and reverence for God help us keep up our physical, emotional, and spiritual health. **Authentic faith**, as the Bible defines it, **means "being sure of what we hope for and certain of what we do not see" (Hebrews 11:1, NIV)**. People who have that kind of faith are less likely to develop medical and mental illnesses or to abuse drugs and alcohol. They are more likely to recover from medical illnesses and surgery. The faithful also tend to have a higher quality of life, which includes strong marriage and satisfaction with one's job and one's life in general. When our lives are grounded in such ways, we have a better chance of staying healthy, or, if we get ill, making a strong recovery.

Perhaps for that reason, religious people tend to live longer than people who aren't religious. The faithful are less likely to engage in risky behavior, and more likely to follow physicians' advice and to engage in healthy behavior, such as exercising, eating a healthy diet, and wearing seatbelts. This thoughtful care for themselves stems from the high value and satisfaction they find in their lives, and their determination to treat the body as the temple God gave them.

Why does religion strengthen our powers to heal, and even protect us from falling ill? In *The Faith Factor: Proof of the Healing Power of Prayer* (Viking, 1998), I give some answers. Religious practice:

1. Lessens the likelihood of depression and strengthens our ability to cope with the stresses in our lives.
2. Reduces drug and alcohol use, and increases willingness to work with doctors and other health care providers.
3. Brings renewed spiritual energy through the beneficial role of adoration, worship, confession, repentance, and forgiveness.

Another way religion benefits us is that it provides us with social support. Worshipping with people to whom we are bound in community, by shared beliefs, rituals, sorrows, and joys, can be a powerful source of personal support. It can help us through our own illnesses, by reminding us that our community is pulling for us, body and soul. And in times of serious illness or bereavement, our spiritual community can ease the demands and burdens on us and create an atmosphere that supports healing.

The community itself can thus become a mediator and an

instrument of healing, and open the path for divine intervention. It can help us hold in mind that an infinite God desires the healing of each individual regardless of race or social situation. You will remember the desperate man, ostracized from his society because of his leprosy, who broke through an astonished crowd and fell on his knees before Jesus, beseeching him, "If you are willing, you can make me clean!" And you'll remember the outcome. Jesus said, "I am willing. Be clean!" and the leper was healed (Mark 1:40–41). That story testifies that the compassionate heart of God intends healing for all persons.

The Apostle Paul writes that "your body is a temple of the Holy Spirit, who is in you. . . You are not your own; you were bought at a price. Therefore, honor God with your body" (1 Cor 6:19 –20). This book will help individuals and congregations honor God not only with worship but also with greater determination to treat the body as a temple of the Holy Spirit.

The Association of Black Cardiologists has been a national leader in recognizing the important role that minority congregations can play in preserving and strengthening the individual and collective health of its members. The trust and esteem the church enjoys in the African-American community has helped promote better health for Black Americans—a project very badly needed.

A Minute for Your Health, intended for distribution as part of weekly programs of worship, recognizes the unique importance of the Black church in enhancing the health of African-Americans. While we are among the most deeply religious groups in the United States, too many of us have poorer health and less access to care than other Americans. Each of the book's seventy-five chapters addresses one important health concern that is relevant to the needs of a congregation.

These brief chapters can't cover everything, but each raises an issue that can be discussed more fully by the congregation's health professionals and clergy, either as part of weekly worship services or through fellowship or educational meetings. Health tips provided by A *Minute for Your Health* can be included in your church bulletin. Such information can help close the unfortunate and unnecessary racial gap readily obvious in health statistics today. By reading and discussing these health tips with your family and friends you can help spread the good news.

# A MESSAGE FROM THE PRESIDENT OF THE ASSOCIATION OF BLACK CARDIOLOGISTS, INC.

### Malcolm T. Taylor, M.D.

The "A Minute for Your Health" project began in 1988 when Rev. Nathaniel Johnson of the Mount Moriah Baptist Church in York, PA asked Dr. Stephanie Kong to give brief health-related messages during their Sunday morning services. In Rev. Johnson's words, "I want this congregation to be the most knowledgeable and the most healthy in Pennsylvania." In addition to these brief oral health messages, Dr. Kong wrote them out and published them in the church bulletin so church members could later refer to them.

The Kongs left York, PA in 1991 and relocated in Sacramento, California, where Dr. Stephanie Kong continued this work by having these messages published weekly in the *Sacramento Observer* and encouraged churches to clip these weekly messages and reprint them in their church bulletin.

In 1995, after moving to Atlanta, and believing that these health-related sound bites were well received, Dr. Kong offered them to the ABC and 52 "Minutes for Your Health" were published for the first time under the auspices of the Community

Health Risk Reduction Program Committee of the Association of Black Cardiologists. The objective for each message was to give a minute's worth of health information that members of church congregations can readily understand, accept and use. Ms. Jackie German, who was the Director of Community Programs, helped to prepare the first "Minute for your Health" primer and was particularly instrumental in securing the support of Dr. Dale Mathews, who wrote the foreword.

As you will soon discover, this book is not just about heart disease and stroke. Although both heart disease and stroke are major areas of concern for the Association of Black Cardiologists, we thought it was also important to provide guidance in other areas of health so that our patients, our congregants and peers could begin their journey with the Seven Steps to Good Health:

1. Be Spiritually Active
2. Take Charge of Your Blood Pressure
3. Control your Cholesterol
4. Track Your Blood Sugar
5. Enjoy Regular Exercise
6. Eat Smart and don't smoke
7. Manage Your Weight

All of us have tasted the bitter fruit of one of our loved ones leaving us too soon due to a stroke or a heart attack. Such deaths are shocking to those left to mourn, because often we were not aware until too late that our loved one was ill. This lack of awareness of potential health problems is particularly common in the African-American community.

By consciously reading all the messages, you will be amazed how a little bit of information will impact on your overall health and well being. We tend to ignore symptoms because of denial, fear, or mistrust of the health care industry. Black patients often come for help only when their condition is at an advanced stage and treatment is no longer likely to provide a satisfactory result.

If we are to improve the health of African-Americans, and Americans in general, we must all work together. As it is, too many of the people whose strength and experience we sorely need are cut down prematurely by sickness or death. When this happens, our young people miss opportunities to share the experience of wise elders. The result is that too often the young repeat the mistakes of their own parents, instead of being guided to better lives by the wisdom of their elders.

It was my pleasure to invite Dr. Stephanie Kong to serve as editor for this edition. Our heartfelt thanks to Pfizer Pharmaceuticals for providing the funding. We hope you enjoy the improvements and updates of the information. Some of the material was adopted from other publications, including the ABC Epidemiology Center under the auspices of Ms. Melanie Dowdell.

A *Minute for Your Health* provides a series of health tips that, through study and discussion, can break bad health habits that weaken our community. By spreading the word, in your congregation and the community at large, to your family and your friends, you can make a difference that matters profoundly to us as a people.

*Prevention and early diagnosis are the keys to good health. Each of us should be the bearer of that good news.*

# THE POWER OF ONE MINUTE

*Mike Magee, MD*

*Director, Pfizer Medical Humanities Initiative*
*Senior Medical Advisor, Pfizer Inc.*

We have many choices about how we spend the minutes of our lives. However, for one minute each week, I ask that you spend it on health. African-Americans suffer disproportionately from health conditions including heart disease, cancer, diabetes, and stroke. According to the U.S. Department of Health and Human Services Office of Minority Health, in 1999, heart disease was the leading cause of death for African-Americans, followed by cancer. As a leader in the African-American community, you can make a difference. Through the power of a minute, you can inform and educate someone about his or her health.

Thanks to the partnership between the Association of Black Cardiologists and the Congress of Black Churches, you will be able to use A Minute For Your Health to address important health concerns of your congregation. Each of the 75 chapters briefly addresses an important health topic. The book is a perfect starting point for discussion of these crucial health issues in your church, and a great first step towards programs such as educational meetings, health fairs and screenings.

We at the Pfizer Medical Humanities Initiative understand that patient education and empowerment are essential for healthy communities. That is why we are proud to support the

Association of Black Cardiologists in bringing you A Minute for Your Health. As an influential voice in the African-American community, you can raise awareness of health education, prevention and treatment. Through your leadership, you can encourage the members of your congregation to address these issues with their medical practitioners. Doing so will help eliminate health disparities in our society.

I encourage you to share the messages in this book with your congregation and other community organizations with which you are connected. A minute a week can make a powerful difference in the health of our nation!

# INTRODUCTION

*Again the word of the Lord came to me, saying, "Son of man, speak to your people, and say to them: 'When I bring the sword upon a land, the people shall designate someone their watchman.*

*'When he sees the sword coming upon the land, if he blows the trumpet and warns the people, then whoever hears the sound of the trumpet and does not take warning, if the sword comes and takes him away, his blood shall be on his own head.*

*'He heard the sound of the trumpet, but did not take warning; his blood shall be upon himself. But he who takes warning will save his life.*

*'But if the watchman sees the sword coming and does not blow the trumpet, and the people are not warned, and the sword comes and takes any person from among them, he is taken away in his iniquity; but his blood I will require at the watchman's hand.'*

*"So you, son of man: I have made you a watchman for the house of Israel; therefore you shall hear a word from My mouth and warn them for Me."*

ෆ Ezekiel 33:1–7

Today, heart attacks, strokes and other cardiovascular diseases continue to lead the nation's list of the Top 10 causes of death. In addition, diseases such as HIV/AIDS, tuberculosis and hepatitis keep spreading, despite our best efforts to stop them. The tragic fact is that for African Americans, all these diseases take an especially high toll.

For people of faith, challenges and even tragedies are best met when we can turn our burdens over to God, and find strength in His blessings and grace. Now, the challenge is the very health of our people, and here, too, the path of faith can lead to healing and strength.

Ezekiel 33:1–7 powerfully explains the role of the watchman. If as watchmen, we see each other suffering and dying from disease and poor health, it is not our duty to alert and educate one another? Could this be done to prevent the pestilence from occurring and spreading?

Each of us must first hear the watchman, and follow his warning that we improve our diets, lifestyles and behaviors. But each of us must also *become* the watchman, by doing what we can to help others. If our brothers and sisters succeed in finding and keeping their good health, we succeed; if they fail, we fail. The burden of ill health rests upon each of us. We *are* our brother's keepers!

It is my hope that a physician, nurse, dentist or other health professional will share these messages weekly with a congregation. The messages may be read aloud as part of the service, printed in the church bulletin, or both. We believe that this program is non-intrusive, and at the same time, reinforces the advice of the member's own physician. It is a simple idea that can significantly improve our collective health status.

*"You don't have to be sick to get better."* Most Americans today know what will keep them healthy and what's likely to make them ill. The difficult part is getting people to make this information work for them. For instance, most of us know that:

1. Smoking will increase our risk of heart disease, cancer and emphysema, but one out of four of us (including physicians) continue to smoke;
3. Too much animal fat in our diets will clog our arteries, but we continue to eat hotdogs, hamburgers, bacon and doughnuts;
4. Too much alcohol will ruin our livers, our relationships, and increase our rate of accidents, but many of us continue to drink too much and at the wrong times;
5. Seat belts can save our lives in an accident, if we wear them regularly; and
6. High blood pressure and elevated cholesterol increase our chance of stroke and heart disease, but one out of three of those affected with these health risks do not have them under medical control.

I hope that these messages will help move your congregation toward greater health awareness, and help move members and their families toward changes that will make them healthier, stronger, less likely to fall ill, and more likely to recover if they are afflicted. The messages are offered in the spirit of health ministry, as lessons that may help our children know their grandparents.

Stephanie H. Kong, M.D.
Editor

For more information on any of the issues we talk about in this book, please write to:

B. Waine Kong, Ph.D., JD
Chief Executive Officer
Association of Black Cardiologists, Inc.
6849 B2 Peachtree-Dunwoody Road
Atlanta, GA 30328
800/753–9222
678/302–4222

You may also visit our website: www.abcardio.org

# A MINUTE FOR
# YOUR HEALTH

# 1

———— ⌒⋎⌒ ————

# CHILDREN SHOULD
# KNOW THEIR GRANDPARENTS
# AND BECOME GREAT
# GRANDPARENTS THEMSELVES

*But Jesus Said, "Suffer little children, and forbid them not, to come*
*unto me: for of such is the kingdom of heaven."*
⌒⋎ Matthew 19:14

Grandparents are a national resource. If we are ever going to solve our social problems, we need grandparents to live longer, healthier lives, and to be available to their grandchildren. Think of a community free of juvenile delinquency, adolescent and unwanted pregnancies, school dropouts and under-achievement. These communities can be realized through the influence of grandparents. A child is only a grandparent away from developing into a happy, well-adjusted, contributing member of society. Children readily defy their parents, but they think twice about upsetting grandma or grandpa. There's authority that children respect.

Grandchildren are also fun. In fact, one grandparent said if she knew that grandchildren were going to be so much fun, she would have had them first. This is your legacy and your immortality. After all is said and done, what you leave behind are your children. So, treat them well. Tell them the stories. Teach them to pray and to be respectful. Just be sure you continue to be available to them.

What's the problem? The problem is, due to heart disease and stroke, too many grandparents leave us even before their grandchildren arrive. Cardiovascular disease is the thief that is robbing African American children of their grandparents. It kills more than half of all grandparents—more than all other causes of death, combined. And the pitiful fact is that heart disease and stroke are preventable. These medical conditions are lifestyle problems. How we live as Americans causes tremendous loss of lives in the fifth and sixth decades of life. It is not dramatic breakthroughs in medicine that will make a difference in our life expectancy. This can only come about when we decide to take responsibility for our health and prevent disease before it happens.

The secret to good health and long life lies in your hands. Every little bit you do will either help you a little or hurt you a little.

# 2

———⌒⌒———

# THE ROLE OF RELIGION
# IN MEDICINE

*Even so faith, if it hath not works, is dead.*
⌒⌒ James 2:17

In some societies, the priest and physician are one and the same person, administering spiritual and physical healing with divine sanction. It wasn't until the 1800's that Americans began to separate medicine from religion and place more emphasis on scientific research to cure diseases. Patients as well as physicians began to rely on science and not faith.

Still, over the past several decades, there has been a broad revival of interest in spiritual healing and religious practice and health. The return to spirituality and religion by patients assists their physical healing. That's accepted today by most physicians and other caregivers. Good studies show, for example, that when patients in an intensive care unit who have had heart attacks are prayed for, they leave the hospital 7–10 days before those who have not been prayed for. On the strength of such studies, religion and spirituality have come to be considered a form of complementary medicine. In another important study, Dr. Robert

Hummer, after analyzing the U. S. Household survey, came to the conclusion that African Americans who attend religious services regularly lived, on average, fourteen years longer than African Americans who do not attend.

Much of the research suggests that an active religious commitment is "beneficial for preventing mental and physical illness, improving recovery, and enhancing the ability to cope with illness." Ask any one of the mothers of the church and they will tell you that they don't need studies to confirm the power of prayer. Most people who practice active prayer for healing swear by it.

Some of us aren't surprised to find these living connections between spirituality and healing. One of the original disciples, St. Luke, was a physician, and there are numerous accounts of Christ Himself healing the members of His audience, the relatives of His circle of friends, and strangers that happened upon Him.

God put physicians here to help us also, so you should practice good medical care at the same time you are praying unceasingly that you maintain your health through the power of prayer. God also expects us to take care of His temple by living the kind of life that promotes health. Western medicine and faith can work hand in hand.

Remember that Faith without Works is Dead.

# 3

———cᐱᗡ———

# MORE PREVENTION–
# LESS TREATMENT

*. . . for a man's life consisteth not in the abundance of the things
which he possesseth.*
ᐱᗡ Luke 12:15

Imagine that life is a mountain road that all of us must travel.
Because many of us like to live on the edge, from time to time,
some of us will fall off the precipice and hurt ourselves. Society's
response is to develop a very sophisticated system to respond to our
falling off the precipice. We have a wonderful ambulance system,
trained emergency personnel, great hospitals, and physicians and
surgeons who will pick us up and try to put us back together again.
But wouldn't it make sense to try to prevent the fall in the first
place? What if we just put up some barriers along the way?

That is exactly how we dealt with tooth decay. Not long ago,
everyone expected to gradually replace his or her natural teeth
with false teeth. Many of us even remember toothaches. Dentists
mostly pulled teeth and dental labs were busy making false teeth.
Science provided the answer. They made three recommendations:

1. Fluoridate our drinking water

2. Brush and floss our teeth twice a day
3. See the dentist once a year for check-ups, not just when you have a toothache

It worked! Ninety percent of Americans born in the last forty years will now die with our natural teeth, the denture labs are mostly gone and most dentists now do other things besides pulling teeth. Most of the diseases that plague us are preventable and under our control, we just need to adopt a preventive orientation to life. We can and should prevent bad decisions, debts, unhealthy relationships and disease. We should control the amount of stress in our lives.

Health and wealth go hand in hand. Healthy people tend to be wealthy people because unhealthy people have to spend so much time and resources trying to cure things that should have been prevented in the first place. What is wealth without health?

If we get used to the idea that it is better to prevent a problem or illness than to try to treat it after falling off a cliff, we will live a long time and enjoy a great quality of life. It is very difficult to put Humpty Dumpty together again after a great fall.

As your first step toward prevention as a lifestyle, embrace these "Seven Steps to Good Health" promoted by the Association of Black Cardiologists:

1. Be spiritually active
2. Take charge of your blood pressure
3. Control your cholesterol
4. Track your blood glucose
5. Enjoy regular exercise
6. Eat smart and don't smoke
7. Manage your weight.

# 4

———ᴄᴠᴏ———

# WHAT IS HEALTH?

*. . . for the Lord seeth not as man seeth; for man looketh on the outward appearance, but the Lord looketh on the heart.*
ᴇᴠᴏ 1 Samuel 16:7

The World Health Organization in 1948 defined health as a "state of complete physical, mental and social well-being and not mere absence of disease or infirmity." More and more scientists and doctors add that a state of spiritual well-being is the fourth criteria that should be evaluated when you want to promote health. Taken together, health then becomes a state of complete physical, mental, social, and spiritual well-being. To be truly healthy you have to pay attention to each aspect of your being on a daily basis.

Everyday you should go through a check list to ensure you have made positive strides toward your:

a. *Physical Health*: What are the areas in your physical health that may need your attention—weight loss, control of high blood pressure, exercise, control of your diabetes?

b. *Mental Health*: What are you going to do today to

ensure you protect your emotions and mental health. Did you control your anger, did you laugh today, did you give someone the benefit of the doubt?

c. *Social Health:* What are you going to do today to interact with people and get positive feedback from people? Are you going to talk to friends? Are you going to join a group? How do you interact with the people at work?

d. *Spiritual Health:* What are you going to do to feed your spiritual self? Do your start your day in prayer? Do you meditate? Do you think about what you want from your life and how you might get it? We are spirited beings and regardless of our religious affiliation, it is comforting to know that help is only a prayer away. You never get a busy signal when you call on God.

Give attention to each portion of your well-being each day so that you can be in the best state of health possible.

# 5

----ϭᴠᴢ----

# DO YOU HAVE A
# LIVING WILL AND AN
# ADVANCE DIRECTIVE?

*A good man leaves an inheritance for his*
*children's children.*
ᴦᴠ Proverbs 12:22

A Health Care Advance Directive or Living Will is a document in which you give instructions about your health care if, in the future, you cannot speak for yourself. You can give a family member or friend the power to make health care decisions for you if you cannot make them for yourself. You also can give instructions about the kind of health care you want or don't want.

There is a difference between a Living Will and a Health Care Advance Directive. In a traditional *Living Will,* you state your wishes about whether you want life-sustaining medical treatments if you are terminally ill. In an *Advance Directive* you direct your own care through the instructions you leave, and appoint someone else to make medical treatment decisions for you if you cannot make them for yourself.

If you cannot make or communicate decisions because of a temporary or permanent illness or injury, a Health Care Advance Directive helps you keep control over health care decisions that are important to you. In your Health Care Advance Directive, you state your wishes about any aspect of your health care—including decisions about life-sustaining treatment—and choose a person to make and communicate these decisions for you.

It's important to have an Advanced Directive before you need it because, unless you formally write out your instructions and appoint someone to decide for you, many health care providers and institutions will make critical decisions for you that might not be based on your wishes. In some situations, a court may have to appoint a guardian.

An Advance Directive also can relieve family stress. By expressing your wishes in advance, you help family or friends who might otherwise struggle to decide on their own what you would want done. Be assured that a Health Care Advanced Directive only kicks in if you are unable to make your own decisions.

Every state has laws that permit individuals to sign documents stating their wishes about health care decisions when they cannot speak for themselves. The specifics of these laws vary, but the basic principle of listening to the patient's wishes is the same everywhere. The law gives great weight to any form of written directive. If the courts become involved, they usually try to follow the patient's stated values and preferences. A Health Care Advance Directive is the most convincing evidence of your wishes.

You should immediately do two things:

1.  Appoint someone as your Agent.
2.  Write out instructions for your care.

Stay in control of your own health care! Make your wishes known.

# 6

———— ❧ ————

# WHAT IS A "RISK FACTOR"?

*For if ye forgive men their trespasses, your heavenly Father will also forgive you. But if ye forgive not men their trespasses, neither will your Father forgive you your trespasses.*
❧ Mathew 6:14,15

A risk factor is like running a red light: sometimes you can get away with it, but eventually you are either going to get hit or at least get into legal trouble.

There are specific risk factors for each disease that afflicts humans. A risk factor is a condition that makes it more likely you will come down with a particular disease. Here are some examples:

- Participating in un-safe sexual practices can lead to sexually transmitted diseases such as syphilis, gonorrhea and HIV-AIDS.
- If you don't brush your teeth or you allow babies to sleep with bottles in their mouths, you have increased the risk of developing tooth decay.
- Not washing your hands after you sneeze or use the bathroom is a risk factor for spreading diseases.

- Smoking is a risk factor in causing lung cancer and heart disease.
- Not getting your baby shots increases the risk of developing childhood diseases like whooping cough, measles, and mumps.

Whatever the disease, there are known risk factors that, if avoided, can lead to a healthier, longer life.

Cardiovascular risk factors are those factors that increase the likelihood of your dying at a young age from a heart attack, congestive heart failure, or stroke. The heart and vascular system are affected by risk factors such as being overweight, having diabetes, not exercising or having hypertension. These risk factors are completely controllable by you without you having to go to expensive gyms, having expensive operations, or being on constant diets.

Obesity and diabetes are the greatest risks against your living long enough to enjoy your grandchildren. Sixty percent (60%) of Americans are overweight and another twenty-seven percent (27%) are morbidly obese (meaning over a hundred pounds overweight). When you pack that kind of weight, the fat is stored not only under your skin but also in your muscles—including your heart muscle and your blood vessels. Your heart and blood vessels can't function the way they were intended under this increased strain therefore they suffer damage (heart attacks and strokes).

Obesity also is a risk factor for the development of diabetes. More and more of our teenagers are obese and, therefore, develop cardiovascular diseases in their fourth (4th) and fifth (5th) decades of life. Diabetes can cause your kidneys to fail, your heart to fail, and eventually you die.

Both obesity and diabetes are preventable, so why are Americans continuing their cycle of destruction by eating themselves to death?! Americans spend $100 million dollars per year eating at fast food restaurants, and then spend another $30 million dollars trying to lose weight.

The secret to weight loss is simple and it won't cost you a fortune. You have to burn more calories than you consume. If you want to consume 3,000 calories a day (double the recommended daily caloric intake), you have to make sure you are going to burn 3,000 calories a day. If you don't, then you have gained weight that day. See how simple it is to take control of your life!

Take a minute to write down the health conditions you have, and then write down the risk factors next to each condition. If you don't know the risk factors for a particular condition you have you can call your local health department, your doctor or surf the internet. When you have listed the risk factors, then have a daily routine of attacking each risk factor. If you do that everyday, then you will begin to see results. You can train yourself to eat smaller portions. Just try it and see!

# 7

---cᴧѵ---

# FINDING A MEDICAL HOME

*And thou shalt teach them diligently unto thy children, and shalt*
*talk of them when thou sittest in thine house, and when thou walk-*
*est by the way, and when thou liest down, and when thou rises up.*
ᏇᏗ Deuteronomy 6:7

None of us wants to be homeless. We need a place that gives us
refuge and love, a place among loved ones with whom we can
share the love that gets us through our days. But people often
forget that they also need a medical home—that is, a place
where they:

- Regularly receive the health care they need, and from
  the same caregiver or physician
- Have their medical information stored
- Trust the information being provided to them
- Learn to do what they need to do in order to stay
  healthy.

Your doctor, or other health care provider, home manages your
medical care. Your doctor knows your past medical history,
keeps records, and is alert to any changes in your health. But you

too are an active family member. It is you who must make and keep medical appointments, tell your doctor the whole story about each illness, take your medication, and do what you need to do to stay healthy. It is you who must know what to do in the case of medical emergencies, or if you have an accident or fall ill. If you have a medical home, none of this will be a mystery to you.

Another benefit offered by a medical home is that here you will be given tests you need to take regularly in order to make sure that your body is working as it should—tests like Pap smears, colon tests, mammograms, and blood pressure checks.

Your doctor knows your medical condition and what medications you are using. Your doctor will also catch any sign of an illness at its early stages, when it is most treatable.

Your doctor, who is your primary care provider, needs to know *all* your medical history. So, if you are obliged to go to a specialist, always request that the specialist sends a copy of the results to your primary medical home. It can be dangerous for you if one doctor is prescribing medicine without knowing what another doctor has prescribed. Sometimes you can even fail to get needed treatment because one doctor thinks the other doctor has provided it.

Remember: *"Home is where the Heart is!"* And your medical home is where your health is!

# 8

---ᐳᐸ---

# YOU AND YOUR DOCTOR

*As every man hath received the gift, even so minister the*
*same to another, as good stewards of the manifold grace of God.*
ᐳᐸ 1 Peter 4:10

**It is up to you to have a personal physician to assist you in
maintaining your health or improving your health. You and
your personal physician are in a partnership that requires
trust on both sides!** Usually, if you take active interest in understanding your condition and treatment, that trust comes easily,
out of your good questions and the conversation with your doctor that follows. If you feel that your doctor does not care about
you personally, talk this over with him or her, and if that doesn't
work, find another doctor.

You are entitled to know everything the doctor knows about
you from your physical examination, or any tests that have been
performed on you. Doctors are more than willing to explain
everything to you, if you ask.

Your trust in your doctor can also rest in the assurance that
your doctor is bound by law to keep information you share with
him or her confidential.

If you have to take a new medication or to be hospitalized,

your doctor will probably give you the information you need to understand the treatment. If not, be sure to ask these questions:

- Why am I feeling the way I do? What do you think is wrong with me?
- What will the tests show you and what will you and I do with the results of the tests?
- Do I really need these tests? (You have a right to refuse all tests you deem unnecessary.)
- What side effects will I have with the medication that you prescribed and want me to take? (All medications have potential side effects. You may not have any problems with the medications your doctor wants you to take, but your doctor can predict the side effects you might have.)
- What risks are involved with the treatment you are recommending?
- Do I have any options other than the treatment being recommended? You have a right to know all your options and to choose the option that you believe is best for you.
- How do the benefits of my treatment compare with the risks?
- How is this treatment likely to affect the quality of my life? (Beyond side effects, you should know whether your treatment affects how you feel, your memory, your sleeping patterns, as well as how well you get along with others.)
- Do I really need to be in a hospital or can I have the therapy at home? If I need to be in a hospital, how long must I stay there?
- Will I have any limitations on my activity at home? Are there things that I should or should not do, such as exercise?

- What are the signs and symptoms that I should tell the doctor immediately if they appear?
- What signs and symptoms can wait until the next office visit?

The answers to these questions will put you on the road to becoming a much healthier patient. Your doctor will be happy to cooperate. This is why it's so important that you ensure that you have one medical home and that all your medical information gets there.

# 9

———⚬⌇⚬———

# MANAGED CARE AND YOU

*He that is void of wisdom despiseth his neighbor:*
*but a man of understanding holdeth his peace.*
⚬⌇ Proverbs 11:12

You owe it to yourself to understand managed care so that you can maximize your benefits.

First, what managed care is *not*. Managed care is not an attempt to ration care or withhold care from consumers. Managed care companies are required by law to approve and pay for all medically necessary services that are listed as benefits in your contract with them.

In order for managed care to work for you, you as the consumer must be aware that:

- Your employer, Medicaid, or Medicare, has made a decision concerning benefits to which you are entitled. *It is your responsibility to know what coverage has been purchased on your behalf.* You must also understand that the managed care company will pay only for those benefits that have been purchased for you by your employer, Medicaid, or Medicare. For example, you and your doctor may feel that you need cosmetic surgery. Cosmetic surgery is usually not a covered benefit that your employer, Medicaid, or Medicare pays for. Therefore, the managed care company will not authorize you to receive cosmetic surgery. On the other hand, if the benefit you seek *has* been provided as a covered benefit, then the managed care company must authorize you to have that benefit if the services you seek are medically necessary.

- It is the responsibility of you and your physician to determine with the managed care company whether the services you seek are medically necessary. Often, the outcome will hinge on whether, in your doctor's view, you require a special test or medical procedure to help diagnose or treat your medical problem. Sometimes simpler tests or further observation of your condition is what is needed, rather than an expensive test or surgical procedure. On the other hand, such tests may prove to the managed care company that the more expensive test or procedure *is* needed.

- When you receive services from a physician other than your personal physician, be sure that this physician has a contract with your HMO. When a physician is contracted, you can be sure that his or her credentials are good and that you will not receive a bill for the services performed. When you receive care from non-contracted physicians, you will usually be responsible for payment of the service even when you are a member of the HMO.

Although managed care organizations have many rules and can be a hassle, the benefit to you is to limit what you have to spend from your pocket for health care. This is especially true if you need on-going medication or medical care. Used properly, with the right understanding on your part of the rules of the game, managed care can work for you.

# 10

―――⌒ℑℑ―――

# DID YOU TAKE YOUR
# MEDICINE TODAY?

*For whosoever shall keep the whole law,*
*and yet offend in one point, he is guilty of all.*
ଓ James 1:11

When your doctor prescribes medication for you, it is important
that you take the dosage the doctor orders on the schedule
given. Most medication has limited potency. If your doctor prescribes a medication to be taken four times a day, that usually
means the effect of the medication will probably only last for six
hours, so to get the full benefit, it's important that you take the
medication every six hours while you are awake.

If you have a chronic disease like hypertension, you may
have to take medicines for the rest of your life. Most doctors start
you with one medicine and only add more when your blood
pressure doesn't respond to just one. If you haven't taken the
medication and your doctor doesn't know this, your doctor may
be ready to add more medication, thinking the first one didn't
work.

If you haven't taken your medicine, let your doctor know
why, whether it's because you can't afford the medicine or you

forgot to take it. If you can't afford the medicine, tell your doctor before your leave the office. More often than not, the doctor can give you samples and find other ways to get you the medication you need.

It's also important to take antibiotics until they are all gone. If your doctor prescribed ten (10) days of a medicine and you only take it until you feel better all you have done is killed the weak bacteria. The stronger bacteria need the full ten days to be killed. Sometimes, when you don't kill all of the bacteria, the bacteria can attack vital organs like your heart or kidneys. So it's important that you take all the antibiotic medication that is prescribed for you.

If you have a question about the medication that is prescribed for you, get an answer from your doctor or the nurse. Once you have the information you need, you are more likely to be comfortable with the medication. Invest in your health and take the medication that is prescribed for you.

# 11

---◯ᴧ◯---

# DIE YOUNG AS LATE
# AS POSSIBLE

*Wherefore lay apart all filthiness and superfluity of*
*naughtiness, and receive with meekness the engrafted word,*
*which is able to save your souls. But be ye doers of the word,*
*and not just hearers only.*
ᴄᴏ James 1:21–2

Have you ever wondered why someone you know has a car that looks and acts brand new even though the car is ten years old? Or why someone else has a car less than three years old that looks and performs like a heap of junk? Could it be that the first person just took better care of this expensive property— respected it, was not reckless with it, did not drive it too fast, checked the oil, had it serviced regularly, parked it in a garage, washed it regularly, used only the right fuel, and kept the wheels from banging curbs?

The second person drove the car into the ground (six feet under). He or she did this by never taking it in to be serviced and repaired by the car doctor except when it stopped or made funny noises.

Which one of these pictures fits you?

Not only do many of us treat our cars carelessly, but we also treat our bodies the same way. We don't take our cars in for routine maintenance and don't take the time to do the same thing for ourselves. You've probably heard a friend say, "I can't live without my car. The question your friend should be asking "How well would I live without my body?"

Far too many of us African American people become disabled, get old, or die before our time. We carelessly eat, drink, and smoke, do not exercise, do not see a doctor when we should, and do not follow the doctor's recommendations when we do see one. In the end, we rob God, ourselves, our families, our church, and our communities of an invaluable asset that can't be replaced—ourselves.

It's true that with the human body, as with a car, the product you start with can make a big difference. In most cases, a BMW will last longer than a Chevy, given equal treatment. Similarly, people who are born with good genes are likely to last and stay strong longer than people with bad ones. But most of us come into the world somewhere in between—not with genes that will keep us going no matter how badly we take care of our bodies, and not with genes that will destroy us even if we take the best of care. That's why prevention—taking good care of yourself and seeing a doctor regularly—is so crucial to your health.

Eubie Blake once said, "If I had known I was going to live this long, I would have taken better care of myself."

# 12

————— ⌇ —————

# HEY MOM, DID YOUR BABY GET HER SHOTS?

*He will not allow your foot to slip; He who keeps you will not slumber.*
⌇ Psalm 121:3

Regular checkups at your pediatrician's office or local health clinic are an important way to keep children healthy. During these visits, one of the services that your baby should get is immunizations or baby shots, which provide the best available defense against many dangerous childhood diseases. Immunizations, or baby shots, protect children against: hepatitis B, polio, measles, mumps, rubella (German measles), pertussis (whooping cough), diphtheria, tetanus (lockjaw), *Haemophilus influenzae* type b, pneumococcal infections, and chickenpox. All of these immunizations need to be given before your baby is 2 years old in order for the baby to be effectively protected.

Some moms take their babies to the health department for their baby shots and to the pediatrician for other services. If your baby gets his or her baby shots at the local health department, make sure that you take the baby shot record to the doctor's office every time you go. Giving your baby too many baby shots is just as harmful as not getting the baby shots.

The chart below includes immunization recommendations from the American Academy of Pediatrics. Remember to keep track of your child's immunizations—it's the only way you can be sure your child is up-to-date. Also, check with your pediatrician or health clinic at each visit to find out if your child needs any booster shots or if any new vaccines have been recommended since this schedule was prepared.

*Remember! Always give your baby's doctor the record of baby shots that your child has been given.*

### Recommended Childhood Immunization Schedule United States, 2002

| range of recommended ages | | catch-up vaccination | | preadolescent assessment |
|---|---|---|---|---|

| Age<br>Vaccine | Birth | 1 mo | 2 mos | 4 mos | 6 mos | 12 mos | 15 mos | 18 mos | 24 mos | 4–6 yrs | 11–12 yrs | 13–18 yrs |
|---|---|---|---|---|---|---|---|---|---|---|---|---|
| Hepatitis B | Hep B #1 | only if mother HBsAG (-) | | | | | | | | | Hep B series | |
| | | | Hep B #2 | | | Hep B #3 | | | | | | |
| Diptheria, Tetanus, Pertussis | | | D Tap | D Tap | D Tap | | | D Tap | | D Tap | Td | |
| *Haemophilus influenzae* Type b | | | Hib | Hib | Hib | Hib | | | | | | |
| Inactivated Polio | | | IPV | IPV | | IPV | | | | IPV | | |
| Measles, Mumps, Rubella | | | | | | MMR #1 | | | | MMR #2 | MMR #2 | |
| Varicella | | | | | | Varicella | | | | Varicella | | |
| Pneumococcai | | | PCV | PCV | PCV | PCV | | | PCV | PPV | | |

— — — — — — — — — — Vaccines below this line are for selected populations — — — —

| | | | | | | | | | | | | |
|---|---|---|---|---|---|---|---|---|---|---|---|---|
| Hepatits A | | | | | | | | | | | Hepatitis A series | |
| Influenza | | | | | | Influenza (yearly) | | | | | | |

This schedule indicates the recommended ages for routine administration of currently licensed childhood vaccines, as of December 1, 2001, for children through age 18 years. Any dose not given at the recommended age should be given at any subsequent visit when indicated and feasible. ▉ Indicates age groups that warrant special effort to administer those vaccines not previously given. Additional vaccines may be licensed and recommended during the year. Licensed combination vaccines may be used whenever any components of the combination are indicated and the vaccine's other components are not contraindicated. Providers should consult the manufacturers' package inserts for detailed recommendations.

Approved by the Advisory Committee on Immunization Practices (www.cdc.gov/nip/acip), the American Academy of Pediatrics (www.aap.org), and the American Academy of Family Physicians (www.aafp.org).

# 13

---‹∿›---

# PREVENTION IS
# CHEAPER THAN CURE

*If thou wilt diligently hearken to the voice of the Lord thy*
*God, and wilt do that which is right in his sight, and wilt give*
*ear to his commandments, and keep all his statutes, I will put*
*none of these diseases upon thee.*
⊙ Exodus 15:26

If you were living one hundred or more years ago, you would worry about dying from such diseases as cholera, typhoid, small pox, tuberculosis, scurvy, beriberi and rickets. Today, because of improved nutrition and sanitation, we no longer have to worry about those diseases. Instead, we die of diseases that are a direct result of our "improved" standard of living. Such diseases include:

- Heart attacks
- Strokes
- Cancer
- Accidents
- AIDS
- Cirrhosis of the liver
- Diabetes.

Many of these are preventable.

In the past 100 years, the life expectancy of African Americans has doubled from 35 to 70 years. This longer life span owes to several breakthroughs in knowledge and understanding. Our political leaders helped by cleaning up our sewage systems, purifying our water, and disposing of our garbage. Nutritionists taught us more about healthy diet. Modern medicine taught us about contagious diseases and how to prevent them from spreading. The church taught us that "Cleanliness is next to Godliness."

*Modern medicine has probably taken us as far as it can. We enter a new century where good health depends more and more on the choices we make.* If we want to live longer and to improve the quality of our lives, we must learn to prevent diseases rather than seek cures after we get sick.

Changing the way we live is the best way to prevent disease. The first step is to identify the risk factors in our own lives and take steps to correct them. So here are a few questions you need to ask yourself:

- Are you overweight?
- Do you smoke?
- Do you exercise?
- Do you drink alcohol excessively?
- Do you use street drugs?
- Do you eat much salt and animal fat?
- Do you eat a lot of sugar?
- Do you drink too much coffee?
- Do you drive recklessly?
- Do you have unsafe sex?

If the answer to any of the above is "yes," take stock of yourself and make a change. You are shortening your life and may not experience the full richness of life that is available to you.

Accept the facts: you *are* the master of your body and tomorrow *is* the first day of the rest of your life. When it comes to maintaining your health, you have to be responsible for yourself. You must recognize that there is a cause and effect relationship between what you do and how long we live. Once you have learned to act on this, you can begin to teach it to others.

Let us approach this new century not in quiet desperation but with gusto, each of us fully responsible for our fellow man and for ourselves.

# 14

⸺ ☙ ⸺

# SHOULD YOU PARTICIPATE
# IN A CLINICAL TRIAL

*And Daniel beseeched Ashpenaz to feed the others meat and wine*
*from the King's table but allow Shadrach, Meshach, Abednego and*
*himself to drink only water and eat only fruits and vegetables. At the*
*end of ten days, their countenance appeared fairer and fatter in flesh*
*than all those who ate the King's meat.*
☙ Daniel 1

If you ever made up a new recipe and asked someone to try it, you conducted an experimental trial of your recipe. When pharmaceutical companies think they have come up with a new treatment or a new use for an old compound, they invite a few people to try it before they market it to the general public. In fact, any new soap, deodorant, eye drop, hair treatment, mouth wash or anything that touches or enters the body must be tried on a few people before the manufacturer is given permission to sell it as safe and effective.

If you have ever been given a prescription for the treatment of pain, blood pressure, cholesterol, arthritis, or even the common cold, thank some volunteers who were courageous enough to first try it in a clinical trial before any other human being. The goal of clinical trials is to find better ways to treat and help people.

Historically, mostly white men volunteered for clinical trials. African Americans have been reluctant. Some of the reasons may have had to do with mistrust of the medical system and the doctors conducting the clinical trial, not wanting to be treated like a "guinea pig," or just being afraid. All we can say in answer to these fears is that we've come a long way from Tuskegee, for which we can all be thankful.

Today, the Food and Drug Administration (FDA) sets very high standards of conduct for investigators and the safety of patients who volunteer for clinical trials. Before a drug can be tried in a human being, a study must be approved by a group of community representatives and doctors who monitor the activities of the investigators and assure that each patient is being treated as safely as possible, with dignity and respect. Patients will not undergo any un-necessary or harmful tests and procedures. Most importantly, patients will have every phase of the study explained to them and an informed consent form obtained before they can enroll as volunteers in a clinical trial.

While there can be no guarantees that participating in a clinical trial will help you, there is always a chance that you may receive the most modern and up to date treatment for your condition. Just like your recipe, the results may be better or worse than the old dish you cooked up a long time ago. That's part of the risk of doing a clinical trial. Only you can decide if the benefits to your health are greater than the risks. So, if you are ever invited to participate in a clinical trial, at least talk to the doctor, get the facts, and make an informed decision. Just remember that many other people took a chance when they participated in the clinical trials that now benefit you and your loved ones.

# 15

———⟳———

# WHAT YOU EAT TODAY
# WILL WALK AND TALK
# TOMORROW

*Do not destroy the work of God for the sake of food.*
*All things indeed are pure, but it is evil for the man who*
*eats with offense.*
⟳ Romans 14:20

Americans are malnourished.

How can the richest nation in the world have malnourished citizens? In some parts of the world the most visible sign of malnutrition is that people are thin and emaciated. But people who are overweight are also malnourished. Malnourishment, simply put, is a condition in which a person is not in a good nutritional state; *more is not better!*

For those of us who are overweight, the obvious solution is to *lose weight and get to your ideal weight.* The secret to weight loss is not dieting—it is portion size. *Portion sizes are more important than what you eat! Remember, elephants and hippopotamai are vegetarians—they just eat acres of vegetables each day. Pay attention to your portion size.*

The human body must be in a balanced state of how much

you eat and how much physical activity you engage in. In other words, if you are overweight you must limit the size of the portions you eat *no matter what anyone tells you*, but you must also increase the number of calories you burn through exercise. *You have to be truthful to yourself; if you are a PLUS SIZE person you are NOT in a positive nutritional state and you are putting yourself at risk for a life-limiting event, such as a stroke or heart attack.*

Here are some helpful hints for losing weight:

- *Be true to yourself!* Analyze why you want to lose weight. Is it because it will help you live longer, lower your risk of heart disease and cancer, or because you want to have more energy and feel better? Maybe your motivation is to look more attractive. In any case, you should lose weight because it makes sense to you. You'll only succeed if you're doing this because you *choose* to.
- Discuss with your doctor whether you need to lose weight and how best to do it.
- If you are overweight, you are probably out of shape. You need to exercise. Moderate exercise is helpful if you do it. Don't make the excuse not to exercise because you can't jog or can't afford a gym. You can exercise at home for free and everyone can walk around the block.
- If you decide to lose weight, select a balanced diet that you can maintain and limit your portion sizes.
- Examine your eating habits. Are you eating when you are not hungry, because of social pressure or just because you see or smell food? You should eat only when you are hungry and stop eating when you are full. *Limit your portion sizes.*
- Watch less television! People who watch a lot of televi-

sion are tempted by the abundance of food ads that tempt them to nibble.

- Don't allow any food outside the kitchen and dining room. Don't eat in the bedroom, bathroom, or living room or while watching TV.
- Decide what you are going to eat before you go the grocery store, not after you buy it. If you buy it, you will eventually eat it.
- Shop for food after you have eaten, not when you are hungry.
- Drink a glass of water or eat some fruit before meals and eat slowly. Eating slowly is important because it takes twenty minutes before you *feel* full. It takes your mind that much time to catch up with your body.
- Don't give in to the food pushers in your family. Don't let your mother tempt you with "One little piece of cake isn't going to hurt you" or "I spent the whole day preparing this for you and that's all you are going to eat?" What you eat today will walk and talk tomorrow. Some overweight people only eat 150 more calories per day—that's only one can or bottle of soda!

# 16

—⌀—

# DIABETES: WHAT IS IT AND WHAT CAN I DO IF I HAVE IT?

*. . . Honor shall uphold the humble in spirit*
⌀ Proverbs 29:23

Americans are overweight! Being overweight can and does cause type 2 diabetes or sugar diabetes. Do you remember the Mama in "Soul Food"? Do you remember her burning her arm when she was cooking that good ole soul food, swimming in butter, grease and sugar? Do you also remember that she didn't know her arm was burning? Its because she had type 2 diabetes and one of the symptoms of having advanced type 2 diabetes is that you lose the feeling in your arms, hands, legs and feet because of poor circulation. Mama eventually died in the movie because of uncontrolled type 2 diabetes.

Diabetes happens when the sugar you eat stays in your blood stream and is not carried into the cells. Your organs, your brain, your heart, your kidneys, your blood vessels require sugar to do their work. If the sugar stays in the blood, the blood gets too thick and your brain tells you to drink water to dilute your blood. That's why people with diabetes are thirsty and have to urinate often.

A healthy body moves sugar from the blood to the cells, which is the role of insulin. But the body only makes a certain quantity of insulin. When we eat too much sugar there isn't enough insulin to move the sugar from the blood to the cells, which is why your doctor will put you on insulin. However, the insulin you take as an injection is not as good as the insulin your body makes, and unless you cut down on the sugar you eat, taking insulin will not help you to protect your organs. It is much better to control your dietary intake of sugar, whether your have diabetes or not.

In fact, 30 million Americans are either being diagnosed or on the verge of being diagnosed with type 2 diabetes, as a direct result of overeating. So many Americans are developing type 2 diabetes that this disease was declared by the Centers for Disease Control as the epidemic of our time. If this trend continues, the rate of diabetes will increase by 165% by 2050.

There is hope, however, because even modest lifestyle changes can prevent the onset of the disease or help to control its progression to kidney failure, amputations, blindness, impotence, heart disease, stroke and death. Diabetes is the seventh leading cause of death and 80% of patients with diabetes die from heart disease or stroke.

You don't have to run five miles per day or starve yourself to prevent diabetes. *The commonsense way is just to reduce your portion sizes and the number of calories you take in.* Put another way, you can get into better shape by reducing your diet by the equivalent of one can of soda or a bag of French fries or potato chips, and/or walking a mile each day. This will translate into a better quality of life and a longer life.

It turns out that the difference between a normal person who is not prone to diabetes and an overweight person who pre-

dictably develops diabetes is 150 calories per day, the same calories in a can of coke! Just eating a little less or being a little more
active will reduce your risk of type two diabetes, if you just stick
to your diet program and exercise.

If you develop diabetes it can be controlled. Look at Halle
Berry: she has diabetes but she is also in great shape.
Unfortunately, more diabetics end up as Mama did in "Soul
Food." Let's work together to control the growth of diabetes in
our lifetime.

# 17

———— ✐ ————

# WHAT IS THE
# HEMOGLOBIN A1C TEST?

*. . . For I have learned, in whatsoever state I am,*
*therewith to be content.*
☙ Philippians 4:11

If you have diabetes, you need to make sure your doctor is order-
ing the Hemoglobin A1C test for you at least 4 times a year.
People with diabetes also check the blood level of their sugar
several times a day by pricking their fingers, drawing a drop of
blood, and using a small glucose meter to measure the sugar
level in the drop of blood. This sugar level tells you what is happening with your blood glucose at the time you are measuring
it, but it doesn't tell you what your average blood sugar was for
the past 3 months. The Hemoglobin A1C test, by establishing
the average over a 90 day cycle, lets your doctor see how well
you have been managing your blood sugar. In other words, your
glucose test is a pop quiz and the A1C is a semester exam.

Here's a chart that you can keep with you to tell how well
you are doing with your Hemoglobin A1C.

| HbA1c | Levels | Blood Sugar Level |
|---|---|---|
| 14 | Seriously elevated levels | 360 |
| 13 | | 330 |
| 12 | ———————— | 300 |
| 11 | | 270 |
| 10 | Elevated Levels | 240 |
| 9 | ———————— | 210 |
| 8 | Slightly elevated | 180 |
| 7 | | 150 |
| 6 | ———————— | 120 |
| 5 | Non diabetic levels | 90 |
| 4 | | 60 |

*Remember, when you expose your blood vessels and organs to high levels of sugar for long periods of time, you damage the wall lining to the blood vessels.* Having a high Hemoglobin A1C means you have had high levels of sugar floating around. Damaged blood vessels lead to damaged organs, such as your kidneys, heart, brain and liver.

The Hemoglobin A1C test is the best way to tell how well you are doing at controlling your glucose and insulin levels. If you get a result of less than 7, you are doing well.

# 18

—— ✺ ——

# RECIPE FOR HEALTHY LIVING

*For we walk by faith, not by sight.*
✺ 2 Corinthians 5:7

Here's a simple recipe to promote a healthy lifestyle. If you practice these steps you will experience the fullness and richness in life we all seek.

- 1 ounce of prevention (much better than a pound of cure)
- 5 servings of fruits and vegetables per day
- 8 glasses of water
- A dozen good friends (relatives are okay as well)
- 30 minutes of exercise per day—any kind of exercise
- 4 cups of laughter (no substitutions)
- 1 mustard seed of faith
- 2 tablespoons of patience (add more if you have children)

Add a dash of adventure (fun can be substituted, but increase the amount). Also add a bunch of love (enough to share). Mix well and live long.

The following ingredients are known to ruin your recipe!

- Couch potatoes
- Excessive alcohol
- Smoking
- Stress
- Negative thinking
- Negative attitude
- Excessive fats and sugar in your diet
- Complaining attitude
- Unforgiving spirit
- No social interaction

A wise man once said "As a man thinks, so is he"; truer words were never spoken. What you put into your vessel will bear fruit so make sure that your vessel is getting a good recipe every day.

# 19

———— ∽ ————

# YOU ARE WHAT YOU EAT

*Whether therefore you eat or drink or whatever you do,*
*do all to the glory of God.*
∽ 1 Corinthians 10:31

People who live off their own land and most people in underdeveloped countries have to do a lot of physical labor to get enough to eat. For them, it's no problem burning up everything they eat.

For some of us, however, going to the supermarket is as much physical work as we do. To make matters worse, many Americans also over-eat and do not live in a way that burns off calories.

It doesn't matter what the latest diet fad says; the basic indisputable rule of obesity is, *if we eat more calories than we burn up, the extra calories will turn into fat. If you like to eat, exercise more, burn up the calories. If you do not like to exercise, eat less.*

Most of us eat too much, and the more we eat, the more we seem to need and want. Few of us work hard enough to burn up what we consume. If you insist on eating too much fat, sugar, salt, and calories, you will pay a price. Some foods, like fats, have more calories than other foods. For example, a cup of fat or sugar has twice as many calories as a cup of fruit or vegetables. People sometimes believe that they can't get fat because they are vegetarians. But remember, elephants and hippos are vegetarians.

A calorie is a calorie and it does not matter where it comes from. Most overweight women can lose a pound per week by limiting their calories to 1500 calories a day. Most overweight men can do the same on 1800 calories per day. Just imagine yourself with fifty pounds less weight in just one year. Of course, this also works the other way. If you only gain two pounds per year for twenty years, you will be forty pounds heavier at the end of that time.

To get all the nutrients your body needs, carefully follow a food plan that your doctor or dietician recommends.

The hardest part of any weight loss plan is to admit that your eating habits must change if you want to lose weight. If you can't accept that fact, get comfortable with the likelihood that you will live a shorter, less healthy, and, perhaps, less fulfilling life.

# 20

————— ✴ —————

# HEALTHY EATING LEADS
# TO A HEALTHY LIFE

*And whatsoever ye do in word or deed, do all in the
name of the Lord Jesus."*
✴ Colossians 3:17

Two out of three people will die from cardiovascular disease or
cancer. Eating too much fat contributes to both. Most
Americans, even slim ones, eat too much fat. Why take the risk?
It is time you discovered how delicious low-fat eating can be.

Here are some guidelines for reducing the fat in your diet:

1.  Listen to your body and eat only when you are hungry
    and stop when you are full—no matter how good the
    food is.
2.  Learn to say no to your mother and to all the other fat-
    chefs and fat consumers in your life. They will find
    ways to show their affection for you other than feeding
    you to death. Maybe the time will come when you can
    show *your* affection by leading them toward a healthier
    diet.

3. Find better ways to handle stress than overeating. Take a brisk walk when you feel a binge coming on. You'll find it refreshing, and you'll lose weight.
4. Avoid red meats and eat more fish, fresh turkey and chicken, without the skin and visible fat. But because extra fat and salt are usually added to processed turkey and chicken, a vegetarian diet is even healthier.
5. Use olive, canola, or safflower oils for your gravies when you fry or sauté. Avoid lard, butter, coconut and palm oils.
6. A serving of fruit or raw vegetables before meals will help to fill you up with good stuff and leave less room for the not so good stuff. When you feel that you absolutely have to eat something sweet, try low fat yogurt, sherbet, sorbet, Jell-O, Italian ice, or pudding made with skim milk.
7. Avoid eggnog, mayonnaise, salad dressing, whole milk and cream. Save your two eggs per week for Saturday morning. When you drink milk, make it skim milk, and when you eat cheese, make it low fat, such as cottage cheese, mozzarella, and ricotta.
8. Avoid pastries, doughnuts, and croissants. Eat whole grain bread, English muffins, bagels, pretzels and bread-sticks. Beans (legumes) and cereals are good sub-stitutes for nuts and processed flour.
9. Avoid sausages, scrapple, bacon, hot dogs, hamburgers, and lunchmeats such as corned beef, peperoni and pastrami.
10. Boil, broil, steam, bake and roast, instead of frying.

If you follow these 10 commandments, you will look better, feel better, and live longer.

# 21

———— ⌀ ————

# READ THE LABEL

*As for these four children, God gave them knowledge and
skill in all learning and wisdom and Daniel had understanding
in all visions and dreams.*
☙ Daniel 1:17

If you buy it, somebody is going to eat it. So you need to know
exactly what you're putting into your own stomach or your family's. Knowing the nutritional value of a particular food, along
with ingredients in it that could be harmful, is quite easy.
Thanks to the Food and Drug Administration, the label on the
container of every packaged food you buy lists all the ingredients
in order. By reading the label, you can avoid foods that are bad
for you and enjoy delicious *and* nutritious foods that do you
good.

The label lists the ingredients in their order by weight. If
water is listed first, as in juices and soft drinks, that means there
is more water in it than anything else. If sugar or fat is listed first,
there is more of them than anything else.

For practice, compare the nutritional content of whole milk
to that of skim milk or low fat milk. People have a lot of mis-

conceptions about this. Here are a few facts. Regular whole milk is about 50% fat! Out of 150 calories per serving, 70 calories come from fat. Many consumers believe that 1% milk contains only 1% of the fat that whole milk contains. That's what the dairy wants you to believe. The fact is that in 2% milk, 40% of the calories come from fat, and in 1% milk, 30% of the calories come from fat. Although they are lower in fat than whole milk, by no means are they healthy and low in fat. (Incidentally, in spite of its name, buttermilk *is* low in fat and calories because it gets its thickness from acidification, not from butter.)

Besides telling you all the ingredients, the label lists the percent of the recommended dietary allowance contained in each ingredient, and the types and amounts of fat contained. Finally, the label gives the serving size, number of servings per container, as well as the number of calories per serving.

When the label says, "May contain one or more of the following ingredients," and then lists several oils, it means that the manufacturer has the option of using any of those oils in the product—including coconut and palm oil, which are especially high in fat. When you shop compare similar products and buy those with the lowest fat content.

The FDA has no official definition of "natural," "low cholesterol," "light," "lean," or "low fat," but food manufacturers like to use them, often confusingly. "Natural" does not mean that the ingredients are healthful or that dietary experts approve of them. "All natural ice cream" may contain coconut oil that can raise your cholesterol. Foods low in cholesterol may be high in calories. "Lean" may mean fewer calories but more fats.

Sugars and sweeteners are the most common food additives in American foods and come in many forms—such as dextrose, corn syrup, maltose, and even molasses. Salt is easier to detect because it always has "sodium" in the name—such as sodium bicarbonate or mono-sodium glutamate (MSG).

Be careful about what goes into your body.

# 22

---⌀---

# THE FACTS ABOUT FATS

*Study to show thyself approved unto God, a workman that*
*needeth not to be ashamed, rightly dividing the word of truth.*
☙ 2 Timothy 2:15

All fats are made of saturated, polyunsaturated and monounsaturated fats, in different proportions. Saturated fats, or "bad fats," come mostly from meat and dairy products. Coconut and palm oils are also saturated. These fats raise your cholesterol and clog your arteries. You can recognize them easily because they harden at room temperature.

Less than ten percent of what you eat should come from saturated fats. Saturated fats are commonly found in whole milk, cheese, butter, cream, beef, pork, lamb, and poultry skin.

Marketers of prepared foods high in saturated fats can advertise that they are cholesterol free even if they use coconut and palm oils. But these saturated fats are converted to cholesterol by your body. The truth about coconut and palm oils is that they are naturally high in saturated fat and that you should avoid them.

Once you have reduced the total intake of fats and cholesterol, fine-tune your diet by replacing saturated fats with monounsaturated fats such as olive, canola and peanut oils.

We all have trouble remembering which fats are good, and which are bad. So think of "Poly" and her sisters, "Mono" and "Sat." Polyunsaturated fats are the good fats, which do not harden at room temperature. These include safflower, sunflower, corn, soybean, and cottonseed oils. Also included in this group are fish oils like cod liver oil. Polyunsaturated fats are better for cooking than saturated fats that come from animal fats and tropical oils. There is an even better cooking fat called olive oil, a monounsaturated fat.

There are two types of polyunsaturated fats. Omega-6 fats are the vegetable oils and Omega-3 fats are the fish oils. Whether fat or lean, fish is among the healthiest meats you can choose. Lean fish comes from either fresh or salt water like catfish, trout, perch, and bass, and have little or no Omega-3 fatty acids. But while they don't give you the good fats, they don't give you the bad ones either. Fatty fish usually comes from the deep sea and contain high amounts of Omega-3 fatty acids, which are good for you. The fish highest in Omega-3 fatty acids are sardines, salmon, mackerel and herring.

One warning: avoid shrimp and lobster, which actually contain more cholesterol than most meats.

Except for that, next time you go grocery shopping, "go fish."

# 23

———— ⌀ ————

# "YE ARE THE SALT OF THE EARTH"

*If your brother is grieved because of your food, you are no longer walking in love. Do not destroy with your food the one for whom Christ died.*
⌀ Romans 14:15

*Salt.* This four-letter word packs a punch. It has been used as currency. Man has fought wars over it. Gandhi's resistance to British Rule over India began in resistance to Britain's control of salt.

"Lord, bless the food we are about to eat—and pass the salt." This grace is common in our homes. But for many of us, eating too much salt becomes a health problem.

Why is this substance, so vital to our health, suddenly controversial in our own time? The controversy began when nutritionists learned that by eating less salt we could reduce the risks of water retention and high blood pressure.

The fact is, we now put salt in just about everything we eat and drink. That means we are often getting heavy doses of salt without even knowing it. That's how this simple mineral, which started out as a preservative of food and therefore of life, has become a potential danger for millions of Americans.

Salt contains sodium, one of the "essential elements" that we must eat to survive. Like most other things, if we eat too much of it, it becomes a problem. Too much salt in your body may cause your body to hold on to some of the water it should get rid of. If you have too much water in your system, your blood pressure may go up.

One out of ten of us is said to be "salt sensitive," which means we are more likely to have problems with water retention. Be mindful of the many ways we get excess sodium added to our diet—for example, from:

- Baking soda in baked and canned goods
- Flavor enhancers in canned vegetables
- Meat tenderizers.

Learn to cut down salt in your own kitchen and table. Try substituting garlic, lemon juice, pepper, vinegar and other spices on your shelf. Experiment and try some of those strange-sounding and mysterious spices like paprika, ginger and sweet basil. You may just like it. Or try commercial salt substitutes, which are also high in potassium, an element we need. Since most of us do not eat enough potassium, this is another good reason to try salt substitutes.

# 24

---⌒⌒⌒---

# EXERCISE FOR BETTER
# HEALTH

*Seest thou how faith wrought with his works,*
*and by works was faith made perfect?"*
ᏇᏉ James 2:22

You do not have to be a trained athlete to enjoy the benefits of exercise. A walk around the mall every other day can help burn off excess fat and keep the heart, lungs, muscles and bones in good shape.

Regular exercise improves the way you look and feel, and gives you more of the endurance and energy you need to live an active life. Best of all, it slows down the aging process. Exercise helps keep the body in tune. It improves the circulation in the heart and muscles, and helps maintain the thickness of bones so they will not break so easily.

*Exercise can do more good than any fad diet.* A two hundred-pound woman who wants to lose one pound can do so without cutting down on food if she walks for three miles. At that rate, with a little perseverance and regularity, she can walk herself to a healthier weight.

As if such benefits weren't enough, exercise also helps relieve stress.

When you exercise, drink enough water, especially on hot days. You lose fluids when you exercise, and if you don't replace them, it is possible to get heat exhaustion and heat stroke. *If you are doing vigorous exercise and you feel faint, lightheaded, dizzy, have a headache or feel thirsty, stop at once and drink some water.*

Every so often, we hear about someone who died because he or she had heart disease and over-exerted. You can avoid this by getting a physical exam, and following your doctor's advice about how much and what kind of exercise is right for you. There is no evidence that physically active people are more likely to have heart attacks than inactive people. Just take it easy, and don't overdo it. Little by little you'll get stronger and develop more stamina.

If you *do* feel discomfort in your chest during exercise, stop and contact your doctor. Especially if you have not exercised in a long time. Start slowly and gradually increase how much you do. That way you'll avoid injury to your joints and muscles. Most overweight people only burn up 150 calories less than others.

# 25

———⌀———

# COMMON MYTHS ABOUT
# EXERCISE

*Ye see then how that by works a man is justified,*
*and not by faith only.*
⌀ James 2:24

People resist exercise because they think it will be too hard or because they are overweight. But the fact is, almost anyone can exercise. Twenty to 30 minutes a day is all you need. And one of the best exercises you can do is walking, which is easy, requires no equipment except a good pair of walking shoes, and which most people find very pleasant once they get into it. Each day that you walk, your body becomes a little bit healthier. Before long, you'll also notice that you are becoming stronger and have more endurance. Any day you don't exercise is not a good day.

Here are some common myths about exercise, and some proven truths:

Myth #1: Exercise makes you feel tired. The truth is that as you get in shape, exercising makes you more energetic. Regular exercise can also help you to resist fatigue and handle stress better.

Myth #2: Exercise takes too long. The truth is that tremendous benefits from regular exercise can be achieved with only 20–30 minutes of exercise per day.

Myth #3: All exercise gives you the same benefits. The truth is that, while all physical exercise gives enjoyment, regular and sustained exercise, like walking, jogging, bicycling and swimming have benefits for your heart and lungs. Weight lifting does not have the same benefits as swimming. Actually, lifting heavy weights raises blood pressure. In general, basketball players and swimmers live longer than football players and weight lifters.

Myth #4: The older you are, the less exercise you need. The truth is that we all tend to become less active as we get older. Since everyone can benefit from regular exercise, it is important to sustain a high level of activity even when we are tempted to sit back and rest on our laurels. The important thing is to tailor your exercise program to your ability and fitness level.

Myth #5: You have to be athletic to exercise. The truth is that most exercise does not require any particular skill or training. You simply need to move your muscles vigorously for 20–30 minutes per day. Many people who find organized sports difficult do very well when they find something like walking or dancing that they can excel in.

Commit to something, even if it's simply taking a walk with a friend.
    Just do it!

# 26

---⌒⌇⌒---

# HOW TO REDUCE THE
# STRESS IN YOUR LIFE

*Whom we preach, warning every man, and teaching every man in*
*all wisdom; that we may present every man perfect in Christ Jesus.*
☙ Colossians 1:28

Stress is a fact of life we can't change. But your attitude about
stress can change catastrophe into opportunity. Yes, stress can be
made into a positive experience. Positive stress can provide cre-
ativity to solve problems, energy to perform tasks, or staying
power to get the job done. It can bring out the best in us.

Destructive stress is stress we experience because we feel we
have no control over a situation. Destructive stress helps bring
on heart disease, cancer, ulcers, and many other diseases.

Here is how you can reduce the destructive stress in your life:

- *Have a Positive Attitude!* Alcoholics Anonymous has a
  saying: "Try and think of what was worrying you two
  weeks ago." Most of us can't remember because the
  problem or irritation got fixed. Sometimes our impa-
  tience is what causes the trouble. We may feel we're in
  the middle of a crisis just because we don't know how to

get out of a stressful experience today. So practice patience.

- *Have a plan B.* Know in advance what you will do if your present plan doesn't work. Having a parachute gives you the confidence to take risks.
- *Don't over-commit yourself.* You can't do it all, be everywhere, or be all things to all people.
- *Know your limits.* A day only has twenty-four hours. You can't pack thirty hours into twenty-four hours, no matter how hard you try.
- *Develop the courage to be imperfect and still feel good about yourself.* We all look foolish, sound dumb, and make stupid decisions at times. Making mistakes is a part of living. Only God is perfect.
- *Accept the fact that people will disappoint you, especially your children and others who are special to you.* They are not in this world to live up to your expectations.
- *Don't expect everyone to be fair and reasonable.* Every cloud has a silver lining. Be creative and find it. Even in the best of circumstances there is a down side. But don't curse because roses have thorns. Instead, celebrate because thorn bushes have roses.
- *Just say "No" and mean it.* From time to time, people will make unreasonable demands on you, ask you to do things you do not want to do. You are not in this world to live up to everyone's demands.
- *Accept the fact that things won't always work out the way you want.* Baseball stars make millions of dollars per year and they are lucky to get a hit three out of ten times at bat. Learn to forgive yourself, appreciate and love yourself. After all, that is the greatest love of all.

# 27

⸺◦⌁◦⸺

# HOW TO RELAX

*A cheerful heart is a good medicine, but a downcast*
*spirit dries up the bones.*
෨ Proverbs 17:22

Do you need to settle your nerves? That doesn't have to mean Caribbean islands or expensive spas. Relaxation is a state of mind and of lifestyle. Everyone can relax by just following a few simple rules. That doesn't mean that you'll never feel stressed — only that you'll know how to handle stress, and have fewer occasions to be irritated and short tempered. Here are the rules:

1. Don't purposely put yourself in stressful situations. When possible, avoid situations and people that upset you.
2. Tell yourself a joke. Blow a stressful situation out of proportion to emphasize the absurdity. If you are stuck in traffic, just imagine what it would be like to be stuck there for ten years. By then, your children will be adults and married. If you are lucky, you will miss their teenage years altogether.
3. Sigh a lot and take deep breaths. When you breathe in,

push in on your stomach and hold it in. When you can no longer hold it, let go very slowly.

4. Listen to music you enjoy.
5. Imagine looking at a waterfall and watch your worries wash away. Or imagine yourself as a millionaire, the President, or a knight in shining armor.
6. Walk away from a stressful situation. Take a fifteen-minute walk and swing your arms. As you do, pretend a helium balloon is holding up your head.
7. Talk with friends, but only confide in someone who has your best interests at heart. If you do not have someone to talk to, write a letter to someone or just write out your problems. Talk into a tape recorder if you have one.
8. Make an "appointment" to deal with the problem at another time. Often, you'll find that in an hour or a day, the problem just isn't a problem anymore
9. Take a hot bath—learn from the Japanese, they live longer than anyone else in the world. If you want a quick fix for stress, follow up the hot bath with a very cold shower.
10. Learn to use exercise as stress relief. In any case, move muscle. Play a game, run, skip, and just get out of the house. If you feel violent, take it out on your mattress. Hit it as hard as you want, it will not complain. Avoid watching TV and by all means get out of bed.
11. Alcohol and drugs only make things worse.

On the other hand, by serving others, we receive more than we give away.

# 28

―――― ∽ ――――

# LAUGHTER IS GOOD
# MEDICINE

*For our heart shall rejoice in Him, because we have*
*trusted in His holy name."*
∽ Psalm 33:21

The song says,
When you laugh, the world laughs with you,
When you cry, you cry all alone.

Actually, there is nothing wrong with either laughing or crying.
They are expressions of honest human emotions that can make
you feel less frustrated and less angry. Crying is a way of letting
the hurt out. Even people of great faith, like King David, knew
the power of lamentation. A laugh, on the other hand, is like
sunshine on a cloudy day. Life without laughter is dreary. An
honest laugh cheers us. It is the music, the gospel chorus, of our
conversations. Laughter among friends is the glue that holds
people together. Victor Hugo said, " I like laughter that opens
the lips and the heart, and reveals at the same time, the pearls of
the soul."

In his book, *Laughter is the Best Medicine,* Dr. Norman

Vincent Peale explains that certain disease ailments respond to a healthy emotional attitude, which can be prompted by laughter. A well-known writer has similarly described how he helped himself recover from cancer by watching old Bill Cosby and Flip Wilson videos.

Scientists are now discovering that laughter and a positive attitude can increase the release of endorphins and promote the manufacture of T-cells. Endorphins make us feel good and decrease our sensitivity to pain. T-cells act like sentinels in our blood to remove harmful microorganisms and cells. (Chronic depression can actually weaken your immune system and lower your endorphin level.)

When you laugh, electrical impulses are triggered and chemicals released into your blood stream that dull pain and tranquilize the soul. Other substances that are released with laughter improve digestion, make the blood vessels relax to improve circulation, and lower blood pressure.

A philosopher said over a hundred years ago, "Laughter is the most healthful exercise. It is one of the greatest things that helps the digestion with which I am acquainted. It stirs up the blood, expands the chest, electrifies the nerves and clears away the cobwebs from the brain. It is the cheapest luxury man enjoys."

# 29

―――⌒∿⌐―――

# HOW MUCH SLEEP
# IS ENOUGH?

*We are the new man, which is renewed in knowledge*
*after the image of Him that created us.*
⌒∿ Colossians 3:10

Obviously, we need our sleep. In fact, if you live to be ninety years old, you probably will have spent thirty years of it asleep. Sleep refreshes us and restores our vigor. But no one is sure how that works. The obvious answer would be that our bodies and brains need the rest, but in fact, our brain, organs, and muscles are very much awake twenty-four hours a day.

As you first fall asleep, your brain, along with your blood pressure, heart rate, and body temperature, all slow down and you fall into what is know as *slow wave sleep*. About an hour and a half later, you enter a dream phase, called REM sleep. REM stands for rapid eye movement. Not only do your eyes move rapidly in this phase, but your blood pressure, pulse, and respiration also act erratically. In this state, your brain is as active as when you are awake.

Some people do very well with three hours of sleep and others need ten hours to feel refreshed. It's said that Einstein slept twelve hours a night. Infants sleep up to eighteen hours per day. As we get older, we require less sleep.

Some people can't sleep when they want to. The most common reasons for insomnia are:

- Traveling to a different time zone
- Annoying noises
- Uncomfortable mattresses
- Physical ailments
- Pain
- Drug side effects
- Irregular working hours
- Napping during the day
- Worries, anxiety, and depression.

Some people have trouble falling asleep because of emotional problems that can be corrected with counseling. Still others only imagine that they do not get enough sleep. Under observation, insomniacs often get more sleep than they think they do.

Sleeping pills often make insomnia worse in the end. Most sleeping pills make you miss the most restful sleep cycles and take away your dreams. Don't let anything or anyone take away your dreams! The best ways to improve your sleeping habits are to:

- Avoid naps.
- Exercise during the day so you will be tired at night.
- Avoid watching hyperactive TV shows before you go to sleep.
- Count cows, sheep, or the hairs on the back of your neck
- Learn to meditate

If you still have trouble, talk to your doctor. He or she may help you discover what's keeping you awake, and may also be able to suggest remedies.

# 30

---○ᴧ○---

# CIGARETTE SMOKING AND
# YOUR HEALTH

*Neither give place to the devil. . . .*
ᐎ Ephesians 4:27

Cigarette smoking is addictive and dangerous to your health. Tobacco use is responsible for nearly one in five deaths in the United States—420,000 deaths annually. Smoking and chewing tobacco are major causes of heart disease and many cancers. Smoking may also cause chronic bronchitis and emphysema. During pregnancy, smoking may cause damage to the unborn baby. Children living with smokers have more respiratory disorders, such as bronchitis and asthma.

Passive smoking, which means inhaling someone else's smoke, causes 5,000 deaths a year from lung cancer and heart disease. Besides, smoking:

- Makes your clothes and hair smell awful
- Wrinkles your skin
- Wastes your money
- Makes a chimney out of your nose

- Tells the world that you do not have control over your behavior
- Makes non-smokers stay away from you
- Stains your teeth
- Makes food tasteless
- Makes you cough
- Makes your breath stink. (You miss a lot of hugs and kisses when you smoke.)

If you smoke and want to stop, you should know that people who stop cold turkey are more successful than people who try to stop gradually. It's true that the more you smoke the harder it is to stop, but you *can* stop. You just have to decide to. If you need a little help, your doctor can prescribe nicotine delivered via patches, gum or nasal spray. Some people find it easier to kick the habit by slowly decreasing their dose in this way.

*In just a few years after you stop smoking, your risk of a heart attack declines sharply, to the same level as a non-smoker's.*

You owe it to yourself and your family to give up this addictive drug. We need to train our children not to smoke just as we educate and counsel them on the dangers of other hard drugs.

Remember: The Surgeon General of the United States warns that cigarette smoking is harmful to you and can cause death.

Don't let your life go up in smoke!

# 31

———⌀———

# ALCOHOL MAKES YOU
# A BAD LIVER

*Wine is a mocker, strong drink a brawler;*
*and whoever is led astray by it is not wise.*
ᢒᢦ Proverbs 20:1

A little alcohol per day is not harmful. In the story of the mira-
cle of Canaan, Jesus turned water into wine so the wedding
guests could enjoy themselves. He even suggested that wine
could settle the stomach.

But problems arise when we drink too much. Alcohol can
make us lose control and become abusive. Alcohol is also an
addictive chemical that can be harmful to our health.

In the United States, alcohol consumption has gone down in
the general population. People who drink heavily rely on alcohol for nourishment and lose their appetite for wholesome food,
so they also suffer from malnutrition.

A six-pack of beer or three shots of whiskey a day for ten years
will cause cirrhosis of the liver. *Cirrhosis* describes what happens
to the liver when alcohol or other chemicals cause the normal
tissue to be replaced with scar tissue. At that point, the liver can
no longer do it's job of cleansing the blood.

Cirrhosis of the liver is not reversible. But with good treatment it can be stabilized—*if* the patient stops drinking alcohol and follows a good diet. If you have cirrhosis of the liver, the simple message is to stop drinking and seek medical treatment. If you drink heavily and do not yet have symptoms, STOP while you are still healthy. Why take a chance on this deadly disease?

While we can survive without alcohol, we can't survive without our liver. "With a healthy liver, you can be a long liver, but you can't be a long liver with a bad liver."

# 32

———∽———

# ALCOHOL AND
# YOUR BRAIN

*For the drunkard and the glutton will come to poverty,*
*and drowsiness will clothe a man with rags.*
∽ Proverb 23:21

Alcohol is a major contributor to accidents, drowning, violence, and sexual assaults. There is also good evidence that people who drink too much alcohol are likely to abuse street drugs as well.

Every drink of alcohol destroys brain cells. For moderate drinkers, that loss isn't serious. We have several billion brain cells and we can do very nicely with a few million less. But for an alcoholic, the loss can be critical.

Have you ever had a long talk with someone, but when you say hello the next morning, he or she doesn't remember talking to you? Short-term memory is the first thing to go with alcoholics. Once brain cells are lost, they can never be replaced. Loss of brain cells also hastens senility.

Protect your brain and your brainpower—drink only in moderation.

# 33

―――――⌒ᴠᴏ―――――

# DRINKING AND DRIVING
# DON'T MIX

*Let us walk properly, as in the day, not in revelry and drunkenness,*
*not in licentiousness and lewdness, not in strife and envy.*
⌒ᴠᴏ Romans 13:13

When we think about drinking and driving, the driver is certainly at risk. But there can be more than one victim when a person who has been drinking drives. Drinking alcohol produces poor judgment and slower reaction time. People under the influence of alcohol can feel elated and over-confident. They may drive faster and take risks that they would not ordinarily take. If they take such risks while you're walking or driving near them, you can become a victim.

You can also become a victim by sitting in the passenger seats of a drunk person's car. This advice holds especially true for teenagers and young adults who like to go to bars and stay out late. When Willie Sutton, the bank robber, was asked why he robbed banks, he replied: "That's where the money is." Well, bars are where the alcohol is, and even if the young person is not drinking, he or she will be around many people who are.

Warn your children that they should not drink and drive.

Warn them, as well, that they shouldn't even be in a car with someone who has been drinking. They are at risk of being involved in accident.

Be a friend to your kids, spouse, neighbor and yourself. Join Mothers against Drunk Drivers (MADD). Speak out against mixing drinking with driving.

# 34

———— ⌘ ————

# BUCKLE UP FOR SAFETY

*My people are destroyed for lack of knowledge.*
ᘓ Hosea 4:6

It should trouble us all to see children riding in cars driven by adults, and neither the adult nor the child has a seat belt on. The popular press and television have stressed the importance of seat belts and air bags for the past ten years, yet some Americans foolishly ignore the laws as well as their children's and their own safety.

A car is a 2000–pound weapon. Even at thirty miles per hour, if you have to stop suddenly, anything in the car that is loose becomes a flying object or missile. You may have had the experience of stopping suddenly, so that the purse or grocery bag next to you on the passenger seat hit the floor. Now think of your child sitting or even standing in that seat. If the child isn't protected by a seat belt, he or she will fall to the floor just as the groceries did, or, worse, fly into the windshield.

You need the same protection as your child. If you have to stop suddenly and do not have your seat belt on, your chest will slam into the steering wheel and your head into the windshield.

Car accidents may not be avoidable but such injuries can be avoided.

Here are some common reasons people do not wear seat belts, and the facts these people fail to see:

- *I am not going far.* Most accidents occur within two miles from home.
- *My clothes will wrinkle.* Take off your suit coat while you are driving. In any case, it is better to have wrinkled clothes than to be injured.
- *The shoulder harness chokes me.* Most cars allow you to adjust the shoulder harness.
- *It is okay that my children do not wear seat belts if they are in the back seat.* Princess Diana was in the back seat of her car when it crashed. She died of massive internal bleeding from the impact against the back seat.
- *Wearing seat belts is a hassle.* Recovering from injuries, not to mention funeral expenses, is far more of a hassle.

When you come right down to it, there is no good reason not to wear your seat belt while driving.

# 35

———— ❧ ————

# UNDERSTANDING
# CHOLESTEROL

*We are to be "living sacrifices," holy and pleasing to God—this is our*
*spiritual act of worship. We should also be transformed by the*
*renewing of the mind.*
❧ Romans 12:1–2

We all have cholesterol in our blood. Cholesterol is produced by the liver, and it is necessary to the body because it is part of the outer lining of the cells. But if your cholesterol level gets too high, cholesterol can interfere with the circulation of your blood, preventing oxygen and nutrients from getting to the cells. If your total cholesterol level does get high, you need treatment, which is simple and effective.

Unlike some other dangerous conditions, high cholesterol in itself doesn't cause pain or make you feel tired, weak, or sick. But if you don't do something about it, it can lead to a heart attack or stroke. If everyone in the United States reduced their cholesterol by 20%, the number of heart attacks would decrease by 40% per year.

You can easily find out if you have high blood cholesterol by having a blood test. If is important to know your numbers.

Total cholesterol—less than 200
LDL—less than 100
HDL—more than 60

If your total cholesterol is high, you can lower it by changing the kind of food you eat. The most concentrated sources of cholesterol are egg yolks and organ meats. Cholesterol is only found in animal products—never in plants. But the body can readily convert fats and oils into cholesterol. A diet high in fatty meats and whole milk products stimulates additional cholesterol production.

Some of us will require medication if our "numbers" are abnormally high for one type of cholesterol or another. It a statin or other medication is prescribed for you, these are highly effective treatments, which most likely will become part of your treatment regimen for the rest of your life. Others of us can address our cholestrol issues by exercising more and eating:

1. less saturated fats (hot dogs, hamburgers, sausages and bacon)
2. more fish
3. more fiber (beans, grains, fruits and vegetables)
4. smaller portions

Remember, the knife that you should worry about most is the butter knife.

# 36

———— ৶ ————

# LDL-CHOLESTEROL:
# THE BAD GUYS

*And thou shalt bind them for a sign upon thine hand, and they*
*shall be as frontlets between thine eyes. And thou shalt write them*
*upon the posts of thy house, and on thy gates."*
৶ Deuteronomy 6:8, 9

The bad guy of the cholesterol world is LDL-cholesterol.
Cholesterol is transported in the blood in little packages called
*lipoproteins.* Cholesterol transported by low-density lipoproteins
(LDL) is bad for you. Cholesterol transported by high-density
proteins (HDL) is good for you. When you have too much LDL-
cholesterol moving around in the blood, it spreads like poured
concrete, making a layer of gooey stuff inside the walls of the
blood vessels. This gooey stuff mixes with other substances to
form plaque—a thick, hard coating that can clog the arteries,
especially the small vessels that deliver blood to the heart. The
process is called atherosclerosis.

The more plaque in the arteries, the greater your risk of having a heart attack, because this garbage may eventually completely clog up the arteries. Elevated LDL-cholesterol is considered a reliable predictor of a heart attack. If your LDL number

is more than 100 mg/dl, it is too high. The lower the number, the lower your risk of heart attacks and strokes.

In order to reduce your LDL-cholesterol, eat more fruits and vegetables and reduce egg yolks, red meat and dairy products. And be sure to have your doctor check your LDL levels once a year.

# 37

# HDL-CHOLESTEROL:
# THE GOOD GUYS

*We are vessels of His mercy which He has prepared*
*beforehand for glory.*
   Romans 9:23

If you've ever played PAC-Man, you've enjoyed watching the little head eat up the little dots. HDL-cholesterol gobbles up cholesterol from blood vessel walls and delivers it to the liver where
it is discarded. It picks up the garbage like a good sanitation
worker. A high level of HDL-cholesterol protects against a heart
attack. The opposite is also true—a low level of HDL increases
your risk of a heart attack. Levels less than 60mg/dl contribute to
the highest risk. The higher the better.

Smoking, being overweight, and not getting enough exercise
all contribute to lower levels of HDL-cholesterol. Smokers can
increase their HDL by just stopping their habit. Other ways of
increasing the HDL include eating a healthier diet, losing
weight, and exercising regularly.

Women have protection from heart attack until menopause
because they usually have high HD-cholesterol. Women who

take estrogen hormones after menopause maintain higher levels of HDL-cholesterol than those who do not. Most women should not take hormones though because hormone replacement may increase your risk for certain diseases like breast cancer. Before you go on hormone replacement talk to your doctor.

# 38

---⌒⌒---

# THE DIFFERENCE BETWEEN CHOLESTEROL AND FATS

*Death and life are in the power of the tongue:*
*and they that love it shall eat the fruit thereof.*
⌒ Proverbs 18:21

A food that contains no cholesterol may contain lots of fat. Cholesterol comes only from animal products. But although vegetable shortening, avocado, peanut butter, nuts and coconut oil have no cholesterol, they contain a lot of fat. When you eat too much saturated fat, wherever it comes from, the body converts some of it into cholesterol.

You can help keep your HDL levels high and the LDL levels low by paying attention to the fats you take in. There are three types of fats:

1. Saturated fats, or bad fats, come from animals (lard), coconut and palm oils. Saturated fats harden at room temperature and stimulate the liver to make more LDL-cholesterol.
2. Polyunsaturated fats, or good fats, do not harden at room temperature, and include safflower, sunflower,

corn, soybean, and cottonseed oils. When we substitute these good fats for saturated fat in the diet, the liver makes less LDL-cholesterol.

3. Monounsaturated fats, the best fats, include olive oil, peanut and canola oil. Oils in this group are good for us because when we substitute these for saturated fat they will increase the good cholesterol. Omega-3 fatty acids that come from salmon, sardines, tuna and other fatty fish actually lower total cholesterol and help prevent heart attacks and strokes.

For good health and long life, keep your LDL low and your HDL high!

# 39

———⌒⌒———

# EARLY WARNING SIGNS OF A
# HEART ATTACK

*For God hath not given us the spirit of fear; but power,*
*and of love, and of a sound mind.*
⌒⌒ 2 Timothy 1:7

Every hour, someone in this country dies suddenly from a heart attack. Some of those deaths could have been avoided if the victims or those around them had recognized the early warning signs. By knowing the signs, you can seek help quicker and have a much better chance of surviving the heart attack. Speed is especially important because your brain begins to die if your heart stops for longer than five minutes.

You may be having a heart attack if you experience:

- Dizziness
- Palpitations
- Uncomfortable pressure
- Squeezing
- Pain in the chest lasting more than two minutes.
- Sweating
- Nausea

- Shortness of breath
- Sudden weakness

If you experience any of these symptoms, seek medical help immediately. In most cases, your best first stop is the nearest hospital emergency room. Don't try to drive. Have someone else take you or call 911.

It is normal to deny that something as serious as a heart attack could be happening to you. Too often, people who are beginning to have heart attack symptoms tell themselves it is gas, a sore muscle or fatigue. But you know the signs. Don't take unnecessary chances with your life. Get medical attention at the first sign of a heart attack.

# 40

———ᴄᴧᴐ———

# STROKE
# (BRAIN ATTACKS)

*But be ye doers of the word, and not hearers only,*
*deceiving your own selves.*
ᴄᴧᴐ James 1:22

Some facts about strokes:

- Stroke is the third leading cause of death in the United States
- 500,000 new strokes occur each year
- Hypertension, diabetes, cigarette smoking, heart rhythm irregularities and high blood cholesterol are major risk factors.

Recognize the early warning signs of stroke. Work out with your doctor a good prevention program, including diet and exercise. Early Warning Signs of Stroke include:

- Numbness or drooping of the face
- Weakness of the arm or leg especially on the same side of the body

- Sudden severe, unexplained headache
- Sudden blurred vision
- Unexplained dizziness or falls, especially along with the other symptoms

Remember, most strokes are not painful. If you have any of these "Warning Signs," don't wait! Every second counts in stopping the damage caused by stroke. Call 911

Your medical home can protect you against strokes through prevention programs and, if necessary, prompt and appropriate treatment.

# 41

HARDENING OF THE
ARTERIES

*And when they came out of the boat, immediately the people
recognized Him, ran through that whole surrounding region, and
began to carry about on beds those who were sick to wherever they
heard He was. Wherever He entered, into villages, cities, or the
country, they laid the sick in the marketplace, and begged Him that
they might just touch the border of His garment. And as many as
touched Him were made well.*
ᐂ Mark 6:54–56

*Atherosclerosis* describes what happens when your arteries
become narrowed with plaque: your blood can't freely get
through the arteries to feed the cells that make up your body.

*Plaque* is made up of calcium deposits, cholesterol, and dead
cells. Pieces of plaque can break off and start flowing with the
blood, and clog up smaller arteries downstream. Eventually, this
condition may cause strokes, heart attacks, or kidney failure, and
it can also seriously weaken the blood flow to the legs.

You can prevent atherosclerosis by

- Controlling your weight and blood pressure

- Not smoking
- Cutting back on animal fats in your diet
- Exercising for thirty minutes every day.

Here are some common treatments for atherosclerosis:

1. *Balloon angioplasty.* In this procedure, a surgeon inserts an un-inflated balloon into the clogged artery, and, by blowing it up, squeezes the plaque to the sides of the artery, creating a larger channel for the blood to pass through. Once your artery is opened, the balloon is deflated and pulled out.
2. *Coronary artery bypass* creates new plumbing, using veins taken from the leg to direct blood past the clogged arteries in the heart.
3. *Laser surgery* burns up whatever is blocking the arteries
4. What we can call the rotor-rooter system of surgery lets the surgeon do the same thing a plumber would do with a clogged drain.

Treating atherosclerosis is far better than not treating it. But best of all, avoid it. You can help yourself out by crossing the following items out of your diet:

- Cigarette smoking
- Hamburgers
- Sausages
- Pizza
- Hot dogs
- Doughnuts
- Soft drinks

- Cakes
- Pies
- Cold cuts.

Just doing something that simple, will greatly improve your health and your chances of living a long life.

But prevention is not just avoiding. You can also help keep atherosclerosis under control by exercising daily, and eating more fruits, vegetables, whole grains, and cereals.

# 42

———— ⌒⌒ ————

# INCREASING POTASSIUM
# IN YOUR DIET

*My son, attend to my words; incline thine ear unto my sayings.*
*Let them not depart from thine eyes; keep them in the midst of*
*thine heart. For they are life unto those that find them, and*
*health to all their flesh.*
⌒⌒ Proverbs 4:20–22

Americans eat too much salt and not enough potassium. For good health, we need to keep these two minerals in balance. Potassium helps the muscles maintain their strength. It is also needed by each cell in the body in order for it to do its job efficiently.

Vomiting, diarrhea and certain medications for hypertension, especially water pills, will lower the blood potassium. Low potassium may cause general weakness, (especially in the leg muscles), cramps, and irregular or abnormal heartbeats. A study done at Cambridge University in England found that eating more potassium could reduce the risk of stroke-related deaths by up to 40 percent.

Foods rich in potassium include fish, chicken, beef, beans, green vegetables, and all fruits. Bananas, prunes, cantaloupe, grapefruit, oranges, melons, molasses, potato skins, and berries are particularly good sources. Sun-dried fruits such as raisins, dates, figs, apricots, and prunes are low in sodium and high in potassium.

If you overcook these foods or even just let them sit in water for a long time, the potassium will leach out into the water. If you overcook your vegetables, you will have to drink the "pot liquor" to recover the potassium!

# 43

# PERFORM A DEATH-DEFYING ACT: GET YOUR BLOOD PRESSURE UNDER CONTROL

*And these words which I command thee this day,*
*shall be in thine heart.*
෨ Deuteronomy 6:6

The term *high blood pressure* came into common usage about thirty years ago when researchers began to recognize that it is the number one killer of Americans. High blood pressure (hypertension), because it has no symptoms, is a silent thief that steals someone's friend or relative every minute of every day. This is the number one health problem for African Americans.

To understand high blood pressure, you need to know that all the cells in our bodies need blood rich in oxygen and other nutrients in order to do their work. This enriched blood helps us to move muscles, to taste, to feel, and to stay alive.

As the body consumes energy, it also creates waste. So, the body needs a way to remove this garbage. Picking up the garbage that the cells produce is another job of the heart and the blood vessels (the cardiovascular system). Feeding the cells and removing waste is a big job. To do it, the heart pumps 100,000 times per day every day we live

For reasons we don't fully understand, in one of four Americans, the pressure that pushes blood around the body increases beyond safe limits. If you keep up the pressure on anything, something has to give. In the case of high blood pressure, what usually gives are the vessels that deliver blood to your brain, kidneys, and heart, resulting in strokes, kidney failure, congestive heart failure, and heart attack.

Blood pressure is reported in two numbers. The higher number describes the pressure in the blood vessels when the heart is at work pushing the blood out. This is called the *systolic*. The lower number, the *diastolic*, describes the heart at rest, being filled up with blood. The safe limit for blood pressure is less than 130/85-mm Hg. Numbers above this limit usually require treatment with medicine to reduce the risk of a stroke or heart attack. In general, the lower the number, the lower the risk.

To avoid the consequences of high blood pressure, get your blood pressure checked. If it is too high, see a doctor about it. If you are placed on treatment, follow the doctor's advice, not just for a while but for the rest of your life. Develop a partnership with your doctor to ensure your continued good health.

High blood pressure is one high you do not want. Perform a death-defying act and get your blood pressure under control.

# 44

---◦◇◦---

# CONTROLLING YOUR
# BLOOD PRESSURE

*Then they cried out to the Lord in their trouble. And He saved*
*them out of their distresses. He sent His word and healed them,*
*And delivered them from their destructions.*
◈ Psalm 107:19, 20

Pressure in our arteries is necessary to keep the blood circulating. But when the pressure is too high, there is greater risk that weak sections of our blood vessels will rupture, or that the inside of the blood vessels will become rough, causing clots to develop. The increased pressure also causes the heart to work harder, become larger, weaker, and eventually just give out.

People who have high blood pressure (greater than 140/90-mm Hg) are at greater risk of stroke, heart attack, congestive heart failure, kidney failure, and blindness. The higher the blood pressure, the greater the risk.

The good news is that high blood pressure is easily detected and easily controlled. So get your blood pressure tested. The test is simple, and it may give you longer life.

If you have been diagnosed with high blood pressure:

1. Maintain your ideal weight. If you are overweight, for every three pounds you lose, your blood pressure will go down 2 millimeters of mercury. Every little bit helps.
2. Increase the amount of exercise you do, but follow your doctor's advice about how much exercise is good for you.
3. Reduce the amount of salt in your diet.
4. Keep your appointments with your doctor.
5. Take medication as prescribed by your doctor. Establish a routine for when and where you will take your medication.
6. Check your blood pressure regularly. You may want to do this at home with a device you can purchase at a drug store.
7. If you take blood pressure medicine and experience side effects (such as drowsiness, constipation, coughing or headaches) don't stop your medication, but tell your doctor about the side effects so adjustments can be made.
8. Do not take any prescription medication not prescribed for you, and do not give yours to anyone else.
9. Tell your doctor about all the medications you are taking, including over-the-counter medications such as aspirin.
10. Be sure that you understand when to take your medication—before meals, after meals, on an empty stomach, or before bed.

# 45

---cℐℴ---

# CHILDREN AND
# HEART DISEASE

*We are God's offspring, for in Him we live and*
*move and have our being.*
cℴ Acts 17:28

In general, heart disease affects older people. It's also true that children can handle more junk food than adults without immediate health consequences. But this doesn't mean there are no long-term consequences. The dietary habits of a lifetime begin in childhood, and, for that reason, heart disease starts in childhood, too.

Autopsy studies done on American soldiers killed in Korea and Vietnam showed advanced clogging in their arteries. Most of these soldiers were in their teens and early twenties. Their condition resulted from a diet of hamburgers, steaks, ribs, hotdogs, sausage, and other animal products. On the other hand, autopsies of Korean soldiers who ate mostly vegetables and rice revealed no buildup of plaque or blockage in their arteries. Studies by Dr. Gerald Berenson show that both Black and White children of both sexes had elevated cholesterol and blockage of arteries even at ten years old.

The best time to get our children to eat right and exercise regularly is when they are young. If your children test high for cholesterol, do not panic! You just have to be more conscientious about what they eat. When Guatemalan children were taken off their high vegetable diet and placed on an American diet, they developed elevated cholesterol after just one month. (Do you realize that the filling in Twinkies is made with sugar and lard?) But you can reverse the process just as quickly, by getting your children off French fries, hamburgers, hot dogs and other fast foods (hot dogs, French fries, hamburgers and doughnuts) that can endanger their health.

You talk to your children about not getting into a stranger's car and about looking both ways before crossing the street. It is also time that you talk to them about eating a balanced diet that is low in fats. Remind them that, besides letting them live longer, healthier lives, such a diet will also help their academic and athletic performance and their good looks. That way you appeal to both their intelligence and their sense of self.

Let children of both sexes go shopping with you so you can teach them how to read food labels. Let them cook with you so you can teach them how to discard the skin from chicken, to use olive oil instead of lard or palm oil, and to refrigerate soup and sauces so the fat can be skimmed off. Most importantly, get them to snack on vegetables, pretzels and fruits instead of candy bars, potato chips and cakes. Help them to establish a healthy lifestyle. Good eating is healthy, and fun!

# 46

———◌◊◌———

# CANCER:
# MYTHS AND FACTS

*Your body is the temple—the very sanctuary—of the Holy Ghost, who*
*lives with you, Whom you have received (as a Gift) from God.*
◌◊ 1 Corinthians 6:19

Cancer is the second leading cause of death in the United States, yet only 50% of African American women get pap tests, and only one out of five get regular mammograms, rectal, or breast exams. For the past fifty years, the rate of death from cancer has been decreasing for White Americans but increasing for African Americans.

Some cancers are related to your genes, but several types of cancers can be avoided. What we eat and drink, as well as where we live and work, can decide our fate.

Freedom begins with knowing the facts. Too many of us "know" things about cancer that simply aren't true:

*Myth # 1*
**Cancer is an illness that mostly White people get.**
*Fact*: Cancer death occurs ten years earlier in African Americans than in Whites. An important reason for this is that African

American patients often are not diagnosed early enough. Early diagnosis and timely treatment can make all the difference.

## Myth # 2
### Cancer is fatal. Once somebody gets it, it is over.

Fact: One out of two White Americans who have cancer are completely cured, but only one out of three African American patients are as fortunate. Don't ignore or deny obvious signs and symptoms of cancer. The key to cancer cure is early detection and treatment. Do not wait for pain, because that may be too late.

Here are the signs you must know. See a doctor at once if you have:

1. Been spitting up blood
2. Blood in your stool or if your stool is black in color
3. A mole or wart that changed colors or got bigger
4. Been feeling tired and have lost weight
5. Persistent headaches, blurred vision or weakness in one of your limbs
6. A sore that does not heal
7. Difficulty swallowing, hoarseness, or cough
8. An unexplained lump in any part of your body.

Cancer is a reality for many Americans. Don't get caught up with myths of home remedies. The facts about cancer prevention could save your life. By seeing your doctor for an annual check-up or by sending a loved one to see a doctor if he or she has any of the danger signs we've listed, you help doctors and researchers in their fight against cancer. You may also be saving a precious life.

# 47

⌒∿⌒

# PREVENTING CANCER

*It is neither good to eat meat or drink wine nor do anything by which your brother stumbles or is offended or made weak.*
☙ Romans 14:21

What you put in your mouth has a lot to do with your risk of developing cancer. The American Cancer Society has targeted good nutrition, along with the avoidance of tobacco, as the best ways to prevent cancer. A low fat diet may reduce your risk of breast cancer, and not smoking certainly reduces your risk for lung cancer and other forms of cancer, along with heart disease. Supplementing your diet with vitamin A and E may also reduce your chances of getting lung cancer, and eating foods high in fiber and calcium may prevent colon cancer. By the way, colon cancer is absent in Africa. Why is it so high in African Americans?

Here are the ten recommendations for cancer prevention:

1. Avoid obesity. Overweight people are more likely to get several types of cancer (They are also more likely to get heart disease and diabetes.) For overweight people, weight loss is protection against disease. Your doctor can help you find the weight loss program that works

best for you. (Colon cancer is almot unknown in most of Africa but extremely high among American Americans.)

2. Cut down on total fat intake. Fats should not exceed thirty percent of your diet. Cutting down fat is an effective way to reduce total calories as well.

3. Increase the amount and variety of vegetables and fruit in your diet. Vegetables and fruits contain B-carotene, Vitamin C, and roughage that reduce your chances of stomach, colon and lung cancer.

4. Eat high fiber foods, such as whole grain cereals, vegetables, and fruits. Such foods help move waste products from your colon.

5. Limit consumption of alcohol. Heavy drinkers are at a higher risk of cancers of the mouth, throat, and liver.

6. Avoid smoked, pickled, or nitrite-cured foods. Eating a lot of ham and chemically cured foods can mean a much higher risk of stomach cancer.

7. Do not smoke or chew tobacco.

8. Teach yourself, and your daughters as they reach adolescence, to check for lumps in the breast and have a mammogram every two years if you are over forty or have a family history of breast cancer.

9. Women should get a pap smear annually.

10. Have your doctor check your stool for blood.

Summary: Advancement has been rapid for the early diagnosis and treatment of all tumors. Take advantage of it.

# 48

---⌇---

# LIVING WITH DIABETES

*Let the word of Christ dwell in you richly in all wisdom; teaching*
*and admonishing one another in psalms and hymns and spiritual*
*songs, singing with grace in your hearts to the Lord.*
ᎧᏫ Colossians 3:16

All the cells of the body, and especially the brain cells, need sugar to function properly. The blood releases sugar to the cells when the cells are stimulated by insulin, a hormone produced by the pancreas. When your body does not make enough insulin, or you're loading up on sugar heavier than your insulin can keep up with, you develop diabetes. All types of diabetes (type two diabetes, juvenile onset diabetes, type one diabetes, adult onset diabetes hyperglycemia, or just plain diabetes) occur when the body can't properly store and use "glucose."

One out of four Americans who have diabetes don't know they have it, so it's important for you to recognize the signs. You may have diabetes if

- You are excessively thirsty.
- You urinate frequently.
- You get overly tired for no apparent reason.

- Someone in your family has a history of diabetes.
- You are overweight.
- You have bruises, cuts or infections that just do not heal, and/or you often have an itch.

The more overweight and the older you are, the more likely you are to have this condition.

Diabetes is easy to detect and control, but if you overlook or neglect it, serious consequences—like blindness, sores that will not heal, kidney failure, coma, and strokes—can follow. Treated properly, diabetics continue to feel well and live like anyone else.

Many people control diabetes by taking oral medications. Others require daily injections of insulin. Although insulin treatment is not a cure, conscientious patients can live normal lives with it. Daily injections can supply the missing hormone, though they can't make the pancreas work again.

Besides medication and regular examinations by your doctor, weight management, diet, and exercise are the three best ways to control diabetes. If you are overweight, lose weight. Losing ten pounds will make a big difference by reducing your need for insulin. Exercise is important because, besides helping you keep both your weight and stress down, it helps keep many parts of your body, including your heart and lungs, healthy.

# 49

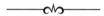

# INFECTIOUS HEPATITIS

*Bless the Lord, O my soul, And forget not all His benefits: Who for-
gives all your iniquities, Who heals all your diseases, Who redeems
your life from destruction, Who crowns you with loving kindness and
tender mercies, Who satisfies your mouth with good things, So that
your youth is renewed like the eagle's.*
Psalm 103:2–5

Hepatitis A is caused by a virus that damages the cells of the
liver. It spreads by close contact either with an infected person
or by drinking or eating foods that contain the virus. It takes two
to six weeks after the exposure for the infected person to get sick.

When hepatitis A strikes, the patient will feel tired, have
stomach pain, lose appetite, feel like vomiting, and generally
feel lousy. The urine may also be as dark as Coca-Cola, and
fever will occur that generally disappears within the first few
days. The most common sign is jaundice, which is a yellowing
of the skin and the whites of the eyes.

If you have these symptoms, contact your doctor immediately. Only a physician will know for sure if you have hepatitis or
not. In the meantime, avoid close contact with others so that you
will not spread the disease.

Children usually develop only mild cases of the disease and get better within one to two weeks. Hepatitis A strikes harder in adults and recovery takes up to six weeks.

If you contract hepatitis, a physician can shorten your recovery period and, possibly, prevent a relapse. The treatment most often requires bed rest and proper diet. In time, you will be as good as new. To prevent the infection in the first place, wash your hands often, avoid close contact with strangers, and be careful about what you put in your mouth.

A public health approach to hepatitis is vaccination for those at risk and gamma globulin injections for those who have been exposed to hepatitis A.

# 50

———— ⚬⁄⁄∘ ————

# ANEMIA

*We then that are strong ought to bear the infirmities of the weak,*
*and not to please ourselves.*
ⓖↈ Romans 15:1

Your body is made up of cells that need oxygen to do their job. If the cells that transfer oxygen are in poor condition, or there are not enough of them to deliver what your body needs, you have what people call "iron poor blood," "low blood count" — or, simply, anemia.

Anemia causes lethargy, dizziness, tiredness and headaches. It occurs when the red blood cells in your body are being destroyed more quickly than they are being made. This can happen because you are not eating the right foods, you are bleeding internally, or your body is unable to make enough red blood cells.

If you have anemia symptoms, consult your doctor. You can also help yourself by eating right. Foods high in the iron and vitamin B12 your blood needs include:

- Fruits
- Whole grain breads

- Beans
- Lean meats
- Fish
- Green vegetables.

People often get low blood pressure and low blood count confused. There is no disease called "low blood pressure." Generally, the lower your blood pressure, the better off you are, if you are not bleeding nor have some other health problem.

*Blood pressure* describes the amount of pressure in your blood. *Anemia* (or low blood count) refers to the quantity of red blood cells in your blood.

Women should get their red blood cell count checked each year when they get a PAP smear. So should anyone with black stool or anyone who has been spitting up blood.

Remember, there is power in the blood.

# 51

———ᴗᴠᴠ———

# STOMACH PAIN

*The Lord is my light and my salvation,*
*whom shall I fear?*
ᴖᴗ Psalm 27:1

Everybody has a painful stomach now and then, because of gas caused by overeating, eating spicy food, drinking alcohol, or just being upset. Stomach pain often goes along with belching, nausea, vomiting, rumbling noises, gas, diarrhea, or constipation. Most of the time it goes away with the help of a little Pepto-Bismol, Rolaids, mint tea, or other antacids, activated charcoal, or the use of a heating pad.

But under certain conditions the pain could be a sign of stomach ulcers, kidney disorders, a urinary infection, appendicitis, hernia, or food poisoning. Here are red light warning signals to watch for:

- Severe pain
- Pain that doesn't go away after using a home remedy
- Pain accompanied by a fever
- Diarrhea
- A burning sensation when you pass water

- Vomiting blood
- Feeling weak

Seek care from your physician if the symptoms above persist. Sometimes a simple call to your doctor can save you a lot of heart ache. If you begin to vomit blood, or you pass out or you begin to see bright red blood in the toilet, this may signal an emergency. If you are at all concerned that you are bleeding call 911.

Bacteria such as E-coli or salmonella, which we can be exposed to if we eat contaminated foods, cause most food poisoning. Both can be present in raw eggs, improperly handled meats, dairy products, seafood, and poultry. Food handlers who do not wash their hands after going to the toilet can also transmit E-coli to food.

E-coli and salmonella take twelve to twenty-four hours before they produce symptoms of stomach pain, vomiting, diarrhea, fever and chill. Such infections usually last for two to three days and are rarely fatal, but it *can* be fatal to the very young and very old. Each year about five hundred infants and old people die from diseases caused by food-borne bacteria.

You can protect yourself by washing with soap and very hot water pots and pans and plates in which you've put raw meats. Thoroughly cook eggs, fish, and chicken before eating them. Eating raw eggs is not a good idea.

Food poisoning can spoil a picnic. Avoid eggs, salad dressing, and dairy products at picnics if they can't be kept cold. Keep hot foods hot and cold foods cold.

Most cases of food poisoning can be treated with bed rest and plenty of tea, activated charcoal tablets, fruit juices, and broth. More serious or persistent cases should be treated by a physician.

# 52

———— ✑ ————

# BREATHING EASIER DURING
# ALLERGY SEASON

*The God who made the world and everything in it; being Lord of
heaven and earth, does not live in shrines made by man, nor is He
served by human hands, as though He needed anything, since He
himself gives to all man life and breath and everything.*
৯৹ Acts 17:24–5

If it's late fall or early spring, it's sneezing time again. But allergy
season doesn't have to be as bad as last year. This time, you will
know how to help yourself feel better.

An *allergy* is an over-reaction that happens when your body
desperately tries to get rid of something you breathed in, such as
ragweed or other pollen; or something you ate; or even something you touched, such as poison ivy. Your body reacts to these
invaders with symptoms such as headaches, itchy eyes, sneezing,
coughing, and skin rashes.

Here are some useful tips about allergies:

- Avoid the things that can trigger your allergies. If you do
  not know what these are, get tested. Your doctor or

health clinic can refer you to someone who can do the tests. If you can't avoid the irritant that triggers your allergy, take antihistamines (Benadryl®, Allerest®, Contac®, Chlortrimiton®, etc.) as directed by your doctor.

- Use an air-conditioner and air cleaner in your home. (But keep in mind, if the temperature gets lower than 70°, it can trigger sneezing.
- If you have a window air conditioning unit, leave the unit off when it is not needed.
- Bright light may trigger sneezing, so wear sunglasses.
- Alcohol can make you more sensitive to allergens (the irritants that trigger the reaction). So, turning down a drink may also turn down your allergies.
- Take allergy medicines before you go to bed, in order to avoid feeling sluggish during the day.
- Don't use Kleenex or paper products to blow your nose—you may be allergic to the paper dust. It is better to use handkerchiefs, but be careful about the detergents and bleaches you use, since you may be allergic to these as well. Double rinsing helps get such ingredients out of your clothes.
- Put a plastic covering over your old mattress or stuffed chair, especially if it has animal fur or feathers, and keep your living environment clean.
- Avoid foods like watermelon, peaches, mangos, or tropical drinks that may make your mouth and throat itch.

In the old days, people with allergies moved to desert climates, where there were few pollens to cause allergies. But today, southwestern states like Arizona are no safer than anywhere else. What happened is that the people who moved there to avoid pollens and grasses ended up putting in golf courses, nice lawns, flowers, and trees. The next time you sneeze or cough, it may not be a cold—it may be allergies.

# 53

———— ∞ ————

# LIVING WITH ASTHMA

*I prophesied as He commanded me, and the breath*
*came into them, and they lived, and stood upon their feet,*
*an exceedingly great host."*
∞ Ezekiel 37:10

Asthma is a disease of the airways in your lungs. About 5 percent of children suffer from asthma, and this rate is increasing. The rate among Latino children under 18 is 7.8 percent; for African American children, 4.2 percent; and for White children, 2.9 percent. The number of children from the inner city who die from asthma has doubled in the last ten years.

Asthma leads to more visits to emergency rooms and absences from school than any other childhood illness. When an asthma attack occurs, the small airways in the lungs close up, plugged with mucous. This blocking of air usually produces a lot of wheezing and coughing, and, in some cases, a life-or-death struggle for oxygen that may last a few minutes but can go on for weeks. Even a short asthma attack can be a frightening experience.

If you or someone you know is prone to asthma attacks, prevention is better than cure. This means you can minimize attacks by learning to identify and avoid irritants like dust and smoke or pollens, or animal dander. If your house is in a neighborhood where the air is especially bad, you may want to get an air filter system. And be sure your furnace filters get changed when they're dirty. Do this for yourself, your children, and your family.

Asthma doesn't have to be a disabling illness. Asthma patients play professional sports, win gold medals at the Olympic games, become successful politicians and scientists, and live very normal lives. The trick is to take the good drugs available to help clear the lungs and airways. Talk to your doctor about them.

The asthma patient can also help her-or-himself by:

- Not smoking or allowing others to smoke around them;
- Exercising regularly;
- Keeping an inhaler within reach at all times;
- Warming up properly before exercise;
- Avoiding things that may cause allergic reactions such as cats, dogs, smoke, dust, pollens, etc.;
- Staying indoors during air pollution alerts;
- Not becoming over-excited and keeping anger in check;
- Not using asthma as an excuse to get sympathy or for not doing things you could but don't want to do;
- Eating sensibly, learning to recognize foods that may bring on an attack, and avoiding fat in your diet;
- Reading and learning as much as you can about the disease, because the more you know, the better able you are to handle problems that may arise.

# 54

# LIVING WITH ARTHRITIS

*And He said unto him, Arise, go thy way:*
*thy faith hath made thee whole.*
 Luke 17:19

Arthritis causes more crippling and discomfort than any other chronic disease, and it affects about 43 million Americans, or one in six of us, of all ages. Every family has elderly members, especially women, who suffer from some form of arthritis. The chief complaints are likely to be about the aching, pain, stiffness, swelling, and tenderness brought on by joint motion.

The most common type of arthritis is osteoarthritis. It results from damage to the ligaments and coverings of the joints in the hands, feet, knees, elbows, ankles and spine. The chief cause is years and years of wear and tear on these joints. That is why it is referred to as "gray hair of the joints." Other causes include injury, hormonal changes, and heredity.

Don't believe the old myths that arthritis patients should not exercise. Aerobic exercise actually reduces joint pain, increases strength and also improves disposition. Try walking, dancing, swimming or bicycling. But be sure to rest your joints if they should become painful.

Surgery is sometimes recommended in severe cases of arthritis to prevent deformities and restore joint function in knees, hips, and shoulders. But for most people, a heating pad, massage, aspirin, and other medication will help. There are a number of splints, braces, and corsets that can also give relief. If you are overweight, losing weight will be a great favor to your joints.

Arthritis can't be cured but, with appropriate medical care, pain and discomfort can be reduced. Talk to your doctor about the best treatment program for you. It may be as simple as aspirin or aspirin-like compounds or your personal treatment plan may be complex. Check with your doctor so that your life with arthritis is manageable.

# 55

—————cᴧɔ—————

# LIVING WITH EPILEPSY
# AND SEIZURES

*Therefore seeing we have this ministry, as we have*
*received mercy, we faint not. . . .*
ᏻ 2 Corinthians 4:1

*Epilepsy* is the medical term for convulsions, seizures or fits. It is
caused by uncontrolled, involuntary activity in the brain.
Typically, a person having a seizure has jerky arm and leg movements, does not respond when spoken to, and, most importantly,
does not remember having the seizure. Not all seizures involve
jerky movements; some seizures just cause the person to stare off
into space. But in both cases, the person will not remember having had a seizure.

Epilepsy can be with you at birth or can be caused by drugs,
alcohol, tumors, injuries or diseases of the brain. Seizures can be
prevented by medications. But most of these medications have
side effects of which patients should be aware.

Treatment of children raises a special problem. Sometimes
children are prescribed Phenobarbital to control seizures.
Phenobarbital can reduce the child's attention span and short-

term memory. But when the drug is withdrawn the child usually regains short-term memory, and whatever negative effects it may have had on his or her ability to think will reverse. Only your doctor should make the decision to withdraw the use of Phenobarbital, so make sure you continue the medication until you and your doctor decide on another course of treatment.

The two most common types of epilepsy attacks are:

*Petit Mal* (little attacks), which usually occur in childhood and stop before twenty years of age. These attacks are characterized by brief periods of inattentiveness or even unconsciousness. These attacks can occur up to 100 times per day and may or may not be followed by Grand Mal seizures.

*Grand Mal* is more common and dramatic. The patient usually loses consciousness and falls, which may result in injury. The patient may also bite the tongue and lose bladder and bowel control.

After the attack, the patient usually falls asleep or feels confused and disoriented. Pain in the stomach and head may follow.

Both children and adults with epilepsy can live normally. Children can do very well at school, and adults can find employment. But children at school and adults on the workplace should select activities or jobs that don't place them around fire, water, machinery or heights.

To prevent seizures from occurring, patients should take their medication as prescribed, get enough sleep, avoid alcohol, and not go for long periods without food.

If you are trying to help someone who has a seizure, place a padded gag between the patient's teeth to keep the airway open and to prevent him or her from biting the tongue. It is also a good idea to restrain the patient to reduce the risk of injury.

Since biblical times, there have been myths and superstitions about epilepsy. But in fact, there is no danger in being around a person prone to epileptic seizures. Most people with epilepsy live normal, healthy lives if they take their medication as prescribed.

# 56

———⌇———

# THE COMMON COLD

*And they that shall be of thee shall build the old waste places:*
*thou shalt raise up the foundations of many generations;*
*and thou shalt be called, The repairer of the breach,*
*The restorer of paths to dwell in.*
⌇ Isaiah 58:12

The average person catches two colds per year. Colds are caused
not by one but by about two hundred viruses grouped together.
A cold starts when a virus penetrates the cells of your lungs and
surrounding tissue. By the time you begin to experience a sore
throat, runny nose, and headache, you may have already had the
cold for several days.

We all tend to catch more colds in winter because the dry
indoor air dries out mucous membranes and lowers resistance
to viruses. We often catch colds from one another. If you touch
the hand of someone with a cold and then touch your own
nose, you're likely to catch the cold. Inhaling droplets from
someone sneezing near you can also infect you. A sneeze has
about 5,000 droplets and can travel across a crowded room for
up to twelve feet.

We know that you can't catch a cold from sitting in a draft, or being exposed to cold temperatures, night air, the rain, or any combination of hot and cold temperatures. You can go out into the cold air immediately after a hot bath without catching a cold. Your child won't catch a cold just by going out into the chill of winter without a coat. He may sneeze from an allergic reaction if he gets his feet in cold water, but he can't catch a cold from not wearing his boots.

As you get older, you are likely to get fewer and fewer colds. Older people develop immunity from previous colds. They are also more careful about germs, so they wash their hands regularly. Babies can get a cold almost every month. Teenagers get about three colds per year. As young people become parents, they will again get frequent colds from their children.

The best way to avoid colds is to eat a healthy diet and take care of your general health, so that your body will be strong enough to fight the virus. Wash your hands three times a day. Get enough sleep. When you become overly tired, you become vulnerable.

If you go to the doctor and take cold remedies, it will take a week to recover. If you do nothing, it will take seven days. There is no cure for the common cold. Cold remedies treat only the symptoms. For instance, anti-histamines will stop only your sneezing.

Should you feed a cold and starve a fever? Actually, you should feed both, even when you don't feel like eating. Any kind of infection will sap your energy, so you need to replenish your calories to keep up your strength. It's actually true that chicken soup is a good food for a cold. It feels good going down and the steam opens your clogged nose.

While you are sick, get plenty of rest, keep warm, drink plenty of fluids, and eat easily digestible foods.

# 57

—◦∿◦—

# TAKE A BITE OUT OF
# TOOTH DECAY

*We are "the sweet fragrance of Christ."*
∾ 2 Corinthians 2:15

Wouldn't it be wonderful if, for the rest of your life, you never had a cavity or a toothache, and never had gingivitis (gum inflammation) or lost a tooth? That can come true if you follow a few simple rules. In a nutshell, brush and floss your teeth daily, and see your dentist once a year.

Teeth decay can cause toothaches when sugars from the food you eat react with the bacteria in your mouth to form an acid. That acid eats away at the enamel on the teeth and causes decay

Many communities have met this problem by adding fluoride to the water. Fluorine hardens teeth and makes them more resistant to decay. But there are also many things you can do for yourself.

Here are ten tips for keeping your teeth strong:

1.  Brush your teeth after each meal, taking care to brush the gums as well as the back and top of the teeth. (If

you prefer, you can massage the gums with a clean finger.) You may even want to lightly brush your tongue and the soft parts of your mouth.

2. Floss your teeth every day. Flossing gets at the plaque that your toothbrush can't reach. Flossing is simple: insert a piece of dental floss between each of the teeth, especially the back ones, and work the floss back and forth against each tooth to remove food particles that promote gum disease.
3. Maintain a good diet with sufficient calcium.
4. Get an annual dental check-up and cleaning.
5. Avoid foods, like sweets, that contain refined sugar.
6. Learn to recognize and treat gum disease quickly. (Gum disease is a major cause of tooth loss).
7. Don't grind your teeth.
8. Don't smoke or chew tobacco.
9. Don't use your teeth to remove caps from bottles.
10. Start your children off right—take them to a dentist before they are five years old, teach them how to brush and floss, and insist they do it daily. You will have to remind them for about five years, but eventually they will develop the routine. The investment will save them pain and suffering, and save you money later.

# 58

---ᐯᐱ---

# DRY EYES

*In whom the God of this world hath blinded the minds of them*
*which believe not, lest the light of the glorious gospel of Christ, who*
*is the image of God, should shine unto them.*
ᐯᐱ 2 Corinthians 4:4

Your eyes are called the windows to your soul, but those windows can get dry and irritated, bloodshot and red, as the result of hay fever, dust, smoke, or foreign particles. Most such irritations are minor, but they can sometimes damage your eyes' delicate tissue. Dryness of the eyes can even cause loss of sight.

Over nine million people describe their eyes as feeling blurry and gritty. Whether you are one of them depends on whether your eyes produce many tears. (Tears are good for the body, as well as the soul.) Some people produce many tears, some do not. The fewer tears you produce, the more irritation you are likely to have.

Older people in particular tend to have dry eyes because the tear glands slow down as we age. Being female also puts you at higher risk of having dry eyes. Living in dry climates can mean trouble too. People who live in Arizona, or other hot, arid climates can brag about their year-round sunshine, but they also have more problems with dry eyes.

Even the way we heat and cool our indoor air can make a difference. Low moisture indoor heating may cause eye irritation. So may air conditioning. In fact, any dry air or wind will tend to dry out your eyes.

Stress plays a role here too. The intense concentration that stress brings about causes us to blink less often, so we tend to have dry eyes in times of stress. Also, when eyelids don't close properly, as in patients with Bell's palsy, dry eyes can be a problem. Dry eyes can also be a side effect of medications like diuretics, antihistamines, beta-blockers, decongestants, birth control pills, and sleeping pills.

You can treat dry eyes with tear replacement drops. There are over thirty types on the market. Experiment to see which one works best for you. One drop in each eye every three hours, whether the eyes feel dry or not, will help. Using such drops can be a preventive act.

Don't use these drops more than five times per day. If you use them too often, the preservative can build up toxins that can damage the surface of the eye. The preservative-free compounds are "Refresh™" and "Ocu-Tears™."

*Don't use anti-redness drops that constrict the blood vessels. They are not the same as tear replacement drops.*

Other options for treating dry eyes are moisture chamber glasses, humidifiers, and even surgery. If the problem persists, talk to your doctor, especially if you wear contact lenses.

# 59

———c╲ɔ———

# FIRST AID

*. . . for I am the Lord God that healeth thee.*
ᘓ Exodus 15:26

If you don't already have a first aid kit in your house, you can make one very easily. Just follow these simple steps:

1. Get a shoebox, old cookie tin, or cigar box, and clean it thoroughly. Label it clearly with the words "First Aid," and make sure every member of your family knows where you keep it.
2. On the inside cover or lid, list the name and telephone numbers of your doctor, the local pharmacy, the poison control center, the nearest hospital, and 911.
3. A basic first aid kit should contain the following items:

- Blunt scissors
- Roll of gauze
- Roll of adhesive tape
- Soap
- Bandages
- Tongue depressor

- Silvadene ointment (for burns)
- Iodine
- Peroxide
- Syrup of Ipecac (to induce vomiting in cases of poisoning)
- 4 X 4 gauze
- Activated charcoal tablets (for food poisoning)
- Tylenol®

Replenish an item when you see it is about to run out.

4.  One member of your family should take the Red Cross First Aid course and be trained in basic Cardio-Pulmonary Resuscitation (CPR).

Here are some helpful first aid hints:

- Clean a cut, and then apply pressure to stop the bleeding.
- If someone swallows poison, call the poison control center before giving Syrup of Ipecac.
- If you suspect that you or a loved one has broken an arm or leg, call the local emergency room for instructions on how to immobilize the limb and how to move the injured person.
- Put cold water or ice on a burn, and call your doctor.

No one plans to have an accident. But you *can* plan how to respond to one.

# 60

—⌇—

# WHAT TO TAKE WITH YOU
# WHEN YOU TRAVEL

*When thou passeth through the waters, I will be with thee; and*
*through the rivers, they shall not overflow thee: when thou walkest*
*through the fire, thou shalt not be burned; neither shall the flame*
*kindle upon thee.*
⌇ Isaiah 43:2

Sometimes, health problems arise while we're traveling. By
doing a little planning ahead, you can avoid some health problems, and, if one does occur for you or a family member, you'll
be sure how to deal with it. Just follow these steps:

1. Be sure you will not run out of your prescription medicines. This means taking enough along with you for the
   length of the trip, or being sure you can renew your
   prescriptions in the places you are traveling to.
2. Drink plenty of fluids and exercise often to keep your
   energy up.
3. Travel can be hard on your stomach. If you're traveling
   abroad, you'll be eating new foods and going through the
   stresses of customs and security. So take along some

antacids—for heartburn, upset stomach, and indigestion.

4. Anti-diarrhea medications or activated charcoal tablets can soothe your stomach, by stopping the cramping and diarrhea.

5. Laxatives can also come in handy. Children sometimes need them. Just eating in a strange place can cause constipation. Kids sometimes go to camp for a week and return home without having had a bowel movement.

6. Antibiotic cream or an antiseptic can help keep little cuts and bruises from becoming infected.

7. An anti-itch cream can help relieve itching caused by insect bites, poison ivy, and rashes.

8. Aspirins or other analgesics come in handy for toothaches, muscle aches, menstrual cramps, arthritis pain, strains, inflammation, and fever.

9. Decongestants relieve nasal congestion and can prevent earaches caused by fluid buildup in high altitudes.

10. Moisturizing cream can help work against the sun and wind, which can dry out your skin. You'll probably be out of doors a lot when you travel, so use sunscreen too. It protects your skin against the damaging effects of ultraviolet light.

11. Eye drops soothe and protect dry, scratchy eyes.

12. An extra pair of eyeglasses is handy in case your regular pair is lost, stolen, or damaged.

13. If you are prone to get motion sickness, take antihistamines. Don't read while in motion, and sit on the left side of planes. Airplanes bank to the right more than they bank to the left.

14. Make sure you have health coverage where you are going, especially if you travel abroad.

# 61

---cho---

# HOW LONG SHOULD
# A PERSON LIVE?

*The days of our years are threescore and ten.*
ᏻ Psalm 90:10

The Bible suggests in Psalms 90 verse 10, that "The days of our years are threescore and ten." This adds up to 70 years. Although there has been a dramatic increase in how long the average person lives, many American don't live to see their 70th birthday.

Too many African Americans, especially African American men, don't live to the biblical age. Life expectancy in the United States for White men is 74, for African American men 66. White women, on average, live to be 80, African American women, 74. Ninety nine percent of us still die before age 85.

In Japan, where people have the longest life expectancy, the average person lives to be 80 years old. The United States ranks seventeenth in the world, and African American men have the shortest life expectancy in the United States. In fact, men in third world countries like Jamaica and Bangladesh live longer than African American men.

There are people who live in isolated parts of the world who have no physicians, hospitals, or synthetic drugs, and yet live longer than we do in the United States. But when they adopt Western lifestyles, they become vulnerable to cancer, heart disease, and stroke.

Regardless of where and how people live, some can drink, smoke, and live dangerously, yet still live into old age. Others come into the world so weak or handicapped that they last only a few days. Most of us fall in the three score and ten years range. But we can live longer if we keep our weight down, exercise, eat wisely, and otherwise live prudent lives. We can guarantee that our lives will be shorter if we smoke, drink too much alcohol, and fail to control our blood pressure.

It's your choice. Choose to get old and not die before your time.

# 62

———◌◌———

# DO THE GOOD DIE YOUNG?

*Our soul waiteth for the Lord: He is our help and our shield.*
◌◌ Psalm 33:20

African Americans die younger than Whites, have more days of disability, and live less healthy lives. Those are the hard facts. Here are some more tips about how to change your life for the better, live longer and healthier, and change statistics in the bargain:

1.  Reduce your stress level. This doesn't mean not working hard. Hard work is good. It means learning how to check your worry and fret over things.
2.  If you don't like your job or other aspects of your life, change them. There are thirteen solutions to every problem.
3.  Learn more skills or improve the ones you have. That increases your options. Become indispensable.
4.  Keep yourself and your family healthy. Healthy people are happier and more prosperous. Poor health is costly, inconvenient, painful and deadly. Only one out of three African Americans regards his or her health as good.

5. Get as much education as you can. Knowledge truly is power. Three times as many African Americans as White Americans have less than a high school education. Only 13 percent of African Americans complete college whereas 70 percent of Whites and 43 percent of Asians finish college.
6. Learn how to resolve conflicts in a way that feels right to both parties. Don't get involved in arguments. Arguments often make enemies.
7. Don't smoke.
8. Drink less alcohol. The rate of liver disease is twice as frequent in African American men than in the general population.
9. Exercise more. Long walks not only help you lose weight but also lower your stress, and, for good measure, help prevent your arteries from being clogged.
10. Obey the rules, if only because not doing so causes you stress. Maybe, you've been getting away with speeding or running stop signs for a while. But you only need to get caught once. That's going to cost you not only money and time, but hassles, inconvenience—and high stress. That's a big price to pay for breaking rules that make sense when you think about them. We spend far too much money on legal fees and fines, and too much time in stress we'd be smarter to avoid.
11. Eat sensibly. Generally, avoid sugar, alcohol, and fats. Take those away, and the rest is likely good for you.

Do not allow your lifestyle to keep you away from your grandchildren.

# 63

---∿---

# THE HEALING POWER
# OF LOVE

*Beloved, let us love one another, for love is of God; and everyone
who loves is born of God and knows God. He who does not love
does not know God, for God is love.*
∿ 1 John 4:7, 9

Love and intimacy affect not only the quality of our lives but our
very survival. Lonely, depressed and isolated people are much
more likely to develop serious illnesses or to die prematurely
than those who keep close ties with friends, relatives, and club,
church and community members. Dr. Dean Ornish, founder of
the Preventive Medicine Research Institute, states that he is not
aware of any aspect of our health—not diet, not smoking, not
exercise, not stress, not genetics, not drugs, not surgery—that
does more to protect us from the likelihood of illness and premature death than the healing power of love and intimacy.
Marvin Gaye was right.

By love, we mean here anything that makes us feel inti-
mately connected with others, part of a community, small or
large. That love can be romantic, but it can also be spiritual or
religious. It works in all things, great and small. We get warmth

from the ties that hold us to other human beings. We get warmth even from the love that goes on between us and a pet, or, sometimes, by just looking up at the sky.

People these days are so caught up in their jobs, their computers, their videos and electronic games that they don't find the time to spend with friends or even family. But spending quality time with friends and family is a necessity, not a luxury. Our need for love and intimacy is as important as eating, sleeping and breathing.

Love comes to those who give it. You can know love by hugging a friend or a child, kissing a mother, embracing a friend. Maybe love means rubbing your father's feet, telling your grandparents that you love them, or writing your brother a letter telling him how much you appreciate him—these are all ways of sharing love. We can spread love by small acts of kindness, such as opening a door for a stranger.

If you aren't experiencing the love you need, know that to love others and be loved, you must first love yourself: the greatest love of all. Start at home and tell yourself how much you love yourself and let your love grow. The world is waiting!

# 64

―――᷍―――

# BREAST FEEDING:
# WHAT EVERY MOTHER
# SHOULD KNOW!

*So, don't be anxious about tomorrow.*
*God will take care of your tomorrow too.*
*Live one day at a time.*
᷍ Matthew 6:34

God has a way of giving every one of us what we need to be
healthy, wealthy and wise. So much so, that in anticipation of
child bearing, He gave every woman two breasts from which
comes the best food your baby can have.

Human milk is healthier for all babies than formula. It is
especially healthy for babies that are born premature or at low
birth weights. Human milk is better for babies for lots of reasons.
Here are some.

a)  Breast milk has helpful antibodies that help children
    fight disease.
b)  Breast milk contains immune cells that fight diseases
    that invade the body through the stomach and
    intestines. When breast milk is swallowed these

immune cells fight disease organisms that might want to invade the baby through the stomach and intestines.

c) Breast-fed babies have lower rates for hospital admissions, ear infections, diarrhea, rashes, allergies and other infections

d) Breast milk promotes development in babies.

e) Breast milk helps the mom and baby bond and provides a nurturing environment.

f) Breast milk helps babies avoid dental caries because the baby isn't left sleeping with a milk bottle in his or her mouth.

A lot more mothers are breast feeding at birth and continue to breast feed up to the child's 6 month birthday. Actually breast-feeding your child to his or her first birthday is recommended. Even if moms go back to work 6 weeks after having their baby, they can breast feed before and after work and provide breast milk for the baby by pumping their breast and storing the milk to be taken by the baby later. You can add solid foods to the babies diet at 4–6 months even when breast-feeding. Preferably, no baby should have cow's milk until they are at least 1 year of age.

Mothers need to remember that whatever they eat or drink will show up in their breast milk, so if a mom is going to breast-feed, she just needs to know what foods she can and cannot eat. Also, every mom who breast-feeds should drink lots of water, which will make the milk come in faster in the beginning, and then keep the milk flowing. Some foods that you can tolerate may give your baby gas or colic. Sometimes it's not clear why a baby develops gas or colic, but that's not a reason to worry. Your diet can be adjusted so that your breastfed baby will have less gas.

Moms on medication can also breast feed. Check with your doctor to see what medications can safely be taken while you breast feed your baby.

Here are some tips for breast-feeding moms:

1. Start nursing your baby within the first hour of delivery. This will help your milk come in and the early milk, called "colostrum" contains helpful antibodies for your baby.
2. Make sure your nipple is as far back in the baby's mouth as possible.
3. Nurse on demand. Don't wake your baby up before your baby is ready. Most breast fed babies want to eat every two to three hours.
4. Babies don't need between meal snacks like sugar water or formula. Your breast milk has all the nutrients the baby needs.
5. Try not to give your baby a pacifier. The sucking required for breast-feeding is different than for pacifiers and may confuse the baby. When babies cry it's usually for a good reason that should be investigated, rather than soothing him/her with a pacifier.
6. Air-dry your nipples after each feeding to make them strong. If your nipples crack, you can put a little vitamin E on them—it won't hurt the baby.
7. Your breast will be full but shouldn't be warm with painful lumps. If your breast develops painful lumps or you get a fever you might have an infection and you should call your doctor.
8. In order to produce milk, moms need plenty of rest, little stress, 6–8 glasses of water a day and a healthy, bal-

anced diet. The average mom only needs to consume an extra 500 calories a day to produce enough milk for her baby–so eat right but not too much!

Above all, enjoy this time with your baby. Time passes quickly and you will treasure forever the memories of this first year of life with your baby.

# 65

---◦◊◦---

# AN ASPIRIN A DAY
# KEEPS THE GRIM
# REAPER AWAY

*For we walk by faith, not by sight.*
◦◊ Corinthians 5:7

Most of us keep a very important medicine in our pocket books, medicine cabinets or on the kitchen counter. The medicine is Aspirin. This drug is widely available, very cheap, and doesn't require a prescription from your doctor. It can save your life if you are having a heart attack.

The symptoms of a heart attack are:

- dizziness
- palpitations
- uncomfortable pressure
- squeezing
- pain in the center of the chest
- sweating
- nausea
- shortness of breath
- sudden weakness

The American Heart Association recommends that anyone having symptoms of a heart attack call 911 and chew a 325 mg tablet (1 adult dose) of aspirin. These two actions will greatly improve your chances of surviving the heart attack.

Aspirin is also effective in lowering your risk of developing a heart attack. Most adults who take one buffered aspirin a day cut their risk of having a heart attack by 50%. When you have your first glass of water in the morning, take your buffered aspirin along with it.

Taking aspirin is no substitute to living the kind of life that promotes good cardiovascular health. Losing weight, exercising and limiting your stress are better than taking that buffered aspirin. However, if you think you are at increased risk for having a heart attack, talk to your doctor and find out if it is okay for you to take an aspirin a day or every other day. Your doctor will know if there are any reasons for you not to take aspirin especially if you are on a blood thinner or have a bleeding ulcer. So check in with your doctor to see if its okay for you to keep the Grim Reaper Away with an Aspirin a day.

# 66

———— ɔʌɔ ————

# BEAT DRUMS,
# NOT EACH OTHER

*Now Cain talked with Abel his brother and it came
to pass, when they were in the field, that Cain rose up
against Abel his brother and killed him.*

ɢ⌣ Genesis 4:8

On average, sixty-five people each day die from interpersonal
violence, and more than 6,000 are physically injured. An estimated 1,000 to 2,000 children die each year from physical
abuse. Violence has a high cost to you, your family and the
nation. The average costs of medical and mental health treatment, emergency medical response, productivity losses, health
insurance, and disability payments for the victims of injuries are
estimated at $34 billion, with lost quality of life estimated at an
additional $145 billion. People who act violently are usually vic-
tims of violence themselves.

There are lots of theories as to why we are violent with one
another. Some people become violent because they want what
you have and feel that they should be able to take it. Some people become violent as a means of making others do what they
want. Sometimes loved ones are violent with each other out of

misplaced passion. One group of people may be violent toward another group in order to exert control. At the base of all violence, however, is frustration.

Whatever the reason, at the root of all violence is selfishness, "I want what I want when I want it." That feeling of false entitlement occurs in violent acts on women at the hands of men, it occurs when one racial group feels it needs to control another racial group, and it occurs when a thief takes what doesn't belong to him.

It will take all of us working together to address the epidemic of violence that exists in our country. One of the practical things we can do is to limit the amount of violence that enters our homes and the minds of our young people through the television, movies and video games. Another thing we can do is to give each other the benefit of the doubt and also forgive each other. A wise man once said, "if a man hits you on one cheek then turn and offer the next check". This is easier said then done. However, each of us can do a little each day to reduce the amount of violence in our lives.

As John Lennon said, "Let's give Peace a Chance."

# 67

———— ᴄⱴᴅ ————

# OVEREATING IN
# CHILDREN

*Wherefore be ye not unwise, but understanding what the will*
*of the Lord is. And be not drunk with wine, wherein is excess,*
*but be filled with the spirit.*
ᴄⱴᴅ Ephesians 5:17, 18

There is a silent predator—call it the obesity demon—that is
making our children fat and unhealthy. Nearly 25% of our children ages 6 to 19 years are overweight; thirty years ago only 4%
of our children were overweight. Being overweight puts our kids
at increased risk of heart disease from high cholesterol and high
blood pressure. It also puts them at risk for Type 2 diabetes,
which was previously considered an adult disease, kidney disease, and some forms of cancer. Just as important, the most
immediate consequence of being overweight is that our children
develop poor self-esteem and depression.

    Obesity in children and adolescents is generally caused by
lack of physical activity, unhealthy eating patterns, or a combination of the two. Genetics can also play a role in determining
a child's weight. But let's concentrate on the lifestyle issues,
since they are the ones we can change and remedy.

Our society has become very sedentary. Television, computer and video games contribute to our childrens' inactive lifestyles. 43% of adolescents watch more than 2 hours of television each day. Children, especially girls, become less active as they move through adolescence. Schools have cut out physical education, and organized sports also suffer in public schools because of lack of funding. Schools have had to put soda and candy machines and fast food restaurants, on their premises to pay for needed equipment and books, which further compounds the vicious obesity cycle. Also, more and more families are turning to fast foods for breakfast, lunch and dinner to meet the demands of having to work and take care of families. African American children often eat high sugar foods (doughnuts and sodas) for breakfast instead of balanced meals from the five (5) food groups. Lack of a balanced meal can produce children who are hyper-active and malnourished.

If your child is overweight, here are some helpful hints:

- Take your child to the doctor to be examined and to define the amount of weight that is desirable to lose.
- Let your child know he or she is loved and appreciated whatever his or her weight.
- Increase the amount of physical exercise your child gets. Make sure your child is physically active. It is recommended that Americans get 30 minutes of physical activity each day.
- Plan family activities that provide everyone with exercise and enjoyment.
- Provide a safe environment for your children and their friends to play actively; encourage swimming, biking, skating, ball sports, and other fun activities.

- Reduce the amount of time you and your family spend in sedentary activities, such as watching TV or playing video games. Limit both activities to less than 2 hours a day.
- Encourage your child to eat when hungry, eat smaller portions and to eat slowly. Eliminate the Supersize mentality.
- Eat meals together as a family as often as possible.
- Carefully cut down on the amount of fat and calories in your family's diet.
- Avoid the use of food as a reward.
- Encourage your children to drink 6–8 glasses of water a day and to limit their intake of beverages such as soft drinks, fruit juice drinks, and sports drinks.
- Stock the refrigerator with fat-free or low-fat milk, fresh fruit, and vegetables instead of soft drinks or snacks that are high in fat, calories, or added sugars and low in essential nutrients.
- Discourage eating meals or snacks while watching TV.
- Eating a healthy breakfast is a good way to start the day, and it may be important in achieving and maintaining a healthy weight.

Your children are your most precious assets and need your protection.

# 68

---cℓ⌒℩---

## SPARE THE ROD,
## SPOIL THE CHILD?

*Provoke not your children to wrath lest they be discouraged.*
ᑫᔆ Colossians 3:21

Disciplining children just got harder, because it is no longer acceptable to "hit them upside their head", beat them with a switch, or shake them the old fashioned way. Children will forever be children and boys will be boys, so their behavior still needs to be corrected so they can succeed in modern society.

Experts disagree on what "good discipline" means today. But there *is* some basic agreement in their thinking. Children need boundaries because they don't know how to set boundaries for themselves. They learn from their parents. So, if they have parents who cannot set boundaries, children grow up with the idea that boundaries are not necessary, even though we live in a society where they will be severely punished if they don't respect these boundaries.

A child's natural inclination is "I want what I want, when I want it," whether it's good for them or not. God provided parents to teach them right from wrong. Most children respond to specific rules and regulations, and to your own counseling as to the difference between right and wrong. On occasion, children specifically disobey their parents. The challenge to parents is how to communicate their authority and their need to be obeyed. Here are some helpful guidelines for discipline that you may want to keep in mind:

- *That which is followed by something pleasureable is likely to be repeated. That which is followed by something unpleasant is likely not to be repeated.* Make specific note of the behaviors you want to decrease and use methods the child doesn't like. This can include turning your back and not speaking. Also make specific note of behaviors you *want*, including doing their homework and responding politely. Smiles, hugs and kisses, even more than money, TV privileges and a "treat," are excellent ways to reinforce the positive behaviors you want to see in your child.

- *Reinforce authority:* Children have to learn to respect all adults and not just their parents. This behavior is essential if the child is to succeed in school. Children should be taught at an early age that adults should be listened to and that they are not equals with adults. A good technique is to train your children to say "Yes, ma'am" or No, sir." Understanding authority is an essential part of success in our society.

- *Keep a cool head:* When disciplining your children, you have to remain in control. Otherwise, the child sees you out of control and decides his or her transgression isn't the issue. You can't trust your judgment when you're angry. Anger leads to impulsive actions and poor problem-solving skills. If you find yourself seeing red, take a time out for yourself. Count to ten (or fifty), and take some good, deep breathes, before you act.

- *Be consistent:* Easier said than done. It is important, though, to enforce your rules consistently. Otherwise, children get a mixed message about whether their behavior is acceptable or not. If you make the mistake of hitting your child just because you are tired and frustrated, the problem will get worse.
- *Be timely:* It's much more effective to respond to a negative behavior immediately after it occurs, rather than use the "wait until your father gets home" response. Denying a child dessert in the evening for misbehavior in the morning is not terribly effective. Do something at the moment to show the child that his or her behavior has consequences.
- *Use age-appropriate strategies:* Your discipline strategies will and should differ, depending on the age of the child. For example, when an 8 month old starts tearing books or chewing on shoes, you can use the technique of remove and distract. Time outs can be used with toddlers. Time-out is literally meant to be "time out from positive reinforcement." That means you select a time-out area that is rather boring (*not* their room full of toys). Time-out should not be done in closets or any place frightening or dangerous for the child.
- *Use repetition and patience:* Discipline doesn't just mean discouraging problem behaviors. It also means encouraging and expecting appropriate behavior. As soon as children learn to talk, we should expect them to say "please" and "thank you."

- *Solicit help from grandparents uncles, ministers and people the child respects.* Gang-up and use group pressure to produce desirable behaviors.

If you follow the helpful hints above there should be no need for spankings. Excessive punishment is not good because children become defensive and just tune out parents. Whatever discipline you use, make sure it matches the transgression, the temperament and age of your child.

# 69

---cハっ---

# CONGRATULATIONS!
# YOU'RE HAVING A BABY!

*Children, obey your parents in the Lord, for this is*
*right. Honor thy father and mother; which is the*
*first commandment with promise.*
ⱺ Ephesians 6:1,2

Having a baby is one of life's greatest pleasures, but it's also a time when a lot will be required of both Mom and Dad, during the pregnancy and after. The most important ingredient in having a healthy baby is a healthy mom. The baby will be exposed to everything the mom exposes herself to, so it is important that pregnant moms get as healthy as possible. Here's why that's so important:

- If the mom smokes, the baby is exposed to smoke and nicotine, which are not good for developing babies.
- If the mom exposes herself to drugs and alcohol, the baby is exposed to the same things, which are definitely not good for developing hearts, brains and other important organs.

- If the mom is under stress then the baby will be exposed to stress, which is definitely not good for the baby.

Babies exposed to unhealthy substances and stress are more likely to leave the womb early and be born prematurely and at lower birth weights. Low birth weight babies and premature babies do not develop as normally as babies born at full term and at a normal birth weight. Moms who overeat during their pregnancy put themselves at risk for developing diabetes, and also for making their babies very large and prone to being overweight

If the Mom eats healthy, exercises and surrounds herself with a stress-free environment that is full of love and caring, the baby will benefit as well. Babies who are read to or who have songs sung to them are more likely to reach development milestones, like walking and talking, at early ages. Babies born to healthy moms are more likely to engage with other people and form those necessary bonds with their moms and dads.

If you decide to become a mom, we suggest you plan for your pregnancy to ensure that your environment and the environment of your baby is the best it can be. Here are some helpful hints:

1. Pick an OB/GYN physician and make an appointment before you become pregnant. You will have to visit this doctor frequently during your pregnancy, and it's important that you and the doctor are comfortable with each other.
2. Have your first pre-natal visit within the first 3 months of your pregnancy, so that your doctor can ensure that you and the baby are all right.
3. During the first 6 months, you will usually see your

doctor once a month; the visits will become more frequent during your last month of pregnancy.

4. During your pregnancy, you should have at least two
   ultrasounds  to make sure that you and your doctor
   know how many babies you are carrying and that the
   baby, or babies, are developing normally.

5. Be sure to eat healthy foods from all five (5) food
   groups, and not gain too much weight.

6. If you begin to retain a lot of fluid in your ankles or are
   having headaches, be sure to call your doctor.

7. If there are any signs of infection, let your doctor know.
   Infections can cause the baby to be born prematurely.

8. Get information on breast-feeding. Remember your
   breast milk is the best milk for the baby.

9. Be sure to get plenty of exercise. Walking helps your
   pelvic muscles stay loose, which will help you during
   labor.

10. Pick a pediatrician and visit that pediatrician before
    your baby comes so that you know what visits will be
    required right after birth.

Congratulations! You're having a baby and a wonderful
experience awaits you.

# 70

---cℳɔ---

# SEX AND
# RESPONSIBILITY

*Do not fret because of evil men or be envious of those*
*who do wrong. For like the grass, they will soon wither . . .*
*Trust in the Lord and do good.*
ɢ Psalm 37:1–3

More and more people are getting sexually transmitted diseases,
and they are getting them at younger and younger ages.
Thirteen and fourteen year olds, without even the basic understanding of safe sex, are engaging in sexual activities and are
being infected with diseases.

Sex is not an activity that should be taken lightly. In fact, sex
does and can kill. It kills not just with HIV/AIDs but in other
ways as well. If you're too young to have a baby, your chance of
severe complications is high.

When our young people have babies as a byproduct of
unprotected sex, they have just committed themselves to responsibilities likely to hurt their education, their ability to make a living, and even their ability to mature. This is why it is so important that we teach ourselves and our children to act responsibly
when we make decisions regarding sexual intercourse.

If we, as parents, carry out our sexual lives irresponsibly, it should be no surprise when our children mimic our behavior, The culture, too, plays a strong role. If our children are bombarded at early ages with sexually explicit videos and TV, they are more likely to experiment with sex at early ages. Children who experiment with sex at younger ages are also then more prone to develop sexually transmitted diseases or become pregnant due to unsafe sexual practices.

We all have the responsibility to approach sex with respect and caution. The marriage environment is an optimal sexual environment, where two people committed to having sex with only each other, are also responsible enough to bring babies into their lives. Sex outside of a monogamous relationship can be fraught with serious consequences. If you decide to have sex outside of a committed relationship, do the responsible thing and wear a condom or have your partner wear a condom. Condoms effectively prevent the spread of gonorrhea, syphilis and HIV.

Be responsible.

# 71

---cᐱᴐ---

# WHAT IS HIV?

*For ye were sometimes darkness, but now are ye light in the Lord;*
*walk as children of light.*
ᏁᏉ Ephesians 5:8

HIV, Human Immunodeficiency Virus, is a virus that attacks our body's ability to fight infection and cancer. This virus has gotten more widespread since the early 1970s, and today it infects about 160,000 Americans.

The good news about this virus is that you can actually prevent yourself from getting it. It's not like the flu virus or common cold virus, which infect large groups of people each year through airborne transmission. The virus known as HIV can only infect you if you let it, through unsafe sexual practices or from infected needles.

You can also get HIV from blood or blood products of persons infected with the HIV virus. Blood banks are now very good in ensuring that all donated blood is free of the HIV virus, so today the virus is rarely transmitted through blood transfusion. People who get blood born HIV usually get it by sharing needles and syringes contaminated by the HIV virus. When IV drug users who have HIV share their needles with other people, those other people are likely to get the HIV virus.

The HIV virus is transmitted through body fluids. Latex condoms are a good barrier for the transmission of HIV during the sex act.

Mothers who are HIV positive will also expose their unborn babies to the HIV virus. Some of these babies go on to develop the HIV infection and AIDS as well, but some babies born to mothers who are HIV positive do not go on to develop AIDS.

You are not likely to become infected with HIV if you avoid unprotected sex and don't share needles.

# 72

———ↄ\\ↄ———

# WHAT IS AIDS?

*Trust in the Lord and He will make your righteousness shine like the*
*dawn, and justice of your cause like the noonday sun.*
ↄ\\ Psalm 57:5–6

AIDS stands for Acquired Immuno Deficiency Syndrome. Too often, an HIV-infected person receives a diagnosis of AIDS after developing one of the diseases associated with the HIV virus. But an HIV-positive person can also be diagnosed as having AIDS without having one of the AIDS related diseases, if the number of T-cells is low. T-cells help fight diseases, and when those cells are low, our bodies can't fight off bacteria, viruses, or cancer cells.

A positive HIV test result does not mean that a person has AIDS. A diagnosis of AIDS is made by a physician using certain clinical criteria, such as the T-cell count and the presence of one of the diseases associated with AIDS.

Infection with HIV can weaken the immune system to the point that it has difficulty fighting off certain infections. These types of infections are known as "opportunistic" infections, because they take advantage of a weakened immune system to cause illness.

Many of the infections that cause problems for people with AIDS, and may be life-threatening, are determined by the health of the immune system. The immune system of a person with AIDS is weakened to the point that medical intervention may be necessary to prevent or treat serious illness.

Today there are medical treatments that can slow down the rate at which HIV weakens the immune system. There are other treatments that can prevent or cure some of the illnesses associated with AIDS. As with other diseases, early detection offers more options for treatment and preventive care.

If you are infected with the HIV virus, it is important to take your medications so that you can slow down the progression of the infection. A stronger immune system will help you enjoy a higher quality of life.

# 73

———— ⌀〇 ————

# WHO SHOULD GET
# A FLU SHOT?

*When you eat of the fruit of your own hands,*
*you will be happy and it will be well with you.*
๛ Psalm 128:2

The flu, caused by a virus, can make you feel really bad. You're
hot one minute, cold the next, your head aches, and your
energy's gone. Some people never get the flu whether they get
the flu shot or not. Others swear by flu shots. Talk to your doctor about your best option.

### What Is the Flu Shot?

The flu shot is a vaccine that protects against the influenza virus.
Like other shots you've had, it helps your body fight infections.
The flu shot contains a small amount of killed flu viruses. The
flu shot won't give you the flu, but those dead viruses are enough
to get your body's immune system ready to fight off the real flu
when it comes around next winter.

## Who Should Get a Flu Shot?

Almost anyone can get a flu shot, but most kids who are healthy don't need it, because even if they get the flu, they'll probably just be sick for a little while and then get better. But there are some kids who may get very sick if they catch the flu, so doctors recommend that these kids get the flu shot. Kids who have *asthma* or other *lung* problems, *heart* problems, *kidney* disease, *diabetes, HIV*, or *sickle cell anemia* should get a flu shot every year.

Another reason to get a flu shot is to protect someone in your family who might get very sick if that person caught the flu. If you live with someone who has any of the medical problems listed above and you get the flu, that person could get very sick. Older people also should get flu shots, because their immune systems (the body's disease-fighting system) aren't as strong.

Babies and little kids can get very sick from the flu, and doctors encourage parents to have their kids who are between 6 months and 2 years old get flu shots. Babies younger than 6 months old also could get very sick from the flu, but they are too young for a flu shot. That means it might be wise, if you're about to bring a new baby into the family, to have everyone in the family get their flu shots. In that way, they help protect the baby.

A yearly flu shot is recommended for the following groups of people who are at increased risk for serious complications from the flu:

- persons aged over 50 years old;
- residents of nursing homes and other long-term care facilities that house persons of any age who have long-term illnesses;

- adults and children 6 months of age or over who have chronic heart or lung conditions, including asthma;
- adults and children 6 months of age or over who need regular medical care or had to be in a hospital because of metabolic diseases (like diabetes), chronic kidney disease, or weakened immune system (including immune system problems caused by medicine or by infection with human immunodeficiency virus;
- children and teenagers aged 6 months to 18 years who are on long-term aspirin therapy and therefore could develop Reye Syndrome after the flu; and
- women who will be more than 3 months pregnant during the flu season.

If you or your family member fits one of the situations listed above you may benefit from the flu shot.

# 74

———— ⌒⌒ ————

# THE TIES THAT BIND –
# THE FAMILY AND ITS
# IMPORTANCE

*And walk in love, as Christ also hath loved us, and hath*
*given Himself as an offering.*
☙ Ephesians 5:2

For a while, when it seemed that America was moving too fast, people stopped talking about the fundamental importance of family values. Today, many of us view the family unit as the best way to promote mental and physical health of each family member, and to promote stable and well-adjusted children. That concensus has become a movement. If you wish to be part of this movement, here are some steps you can take to strengthen your family.

Step 1: *Make sure everyone in your family knows that your family comes first.* Mr. Spock once said, "The needs of the many outweigh the needs of the one". Everyone in your family unit should know that parents will promote the interests of the family as well as the interests of each family member. As children grow up, they need the assurance that their projects and interests are as important as work responsibilities. Promoting everyone's importance will ensure that each member of the family will promote the "Family First" idea.

Step 2: *Promote each other's success.* In promoting the family unit, it's also okay to want to become an individual with interests outside of the family unit. The family becomes the "safe haven" that everyone can retreat to, while learning to be individuals with their own strengths and weaknesses. A wise man once said, "If you have family, friends and God, you may get tripped up or stumble, but you will never hit the ground".

Step 3: *Promote joint decision-making.* When conflict arises, it's important that the family get together to discuss the problems and solutions. An ideal family get together is one where people can say what they really feel, without fear of reprisal. Some families set aside Thursdays as the day the family gets together to discuss individual and collective challenges.

During these weekly meetings, the children and parents could discuss tough issues—with the ground rules being 1) no criticism and 2) everyone promoting problem solving. Whatever method is used, families should set aside specific times to discuss important decisions and problems, with everyone's understanding that although a democratic process is being promoted, the final decision will rest with the parents.

Step 4: *Never give family members broken cookies.* A lot of families put aside the "good" stuff, like best cuts of meats or unbroken cookies, for company. When company came over when you were a kid, maybe mother would break out the fine china. Such behavior is usually justified along the lines that it is always good to put your best foot forward for company. Well, perhaps we need to put our best foot forward for our families as well.

Step 5: *Teach adaptability and an ability to roll with the punches.* There are no set rules that can govern what families will experience in our uncertain times. Financial successes and failures can occur over-night. If you view the family as a unit that lasts forever, what's good for one member is good for the whole.

Step 6: *Be good listeners.* When family members are experiencing difficulties or significant events in their lives, all family members can participate by listening. That's a way of ensuring the person who needs your support that you understand that their issue is important and worth listening to. When you are acknowledged and listened to by the special people in your life, you can't help but feel special, and draw strength from that feeling.

Step 7: *Teach social responsibility.* A wise prophet once said, "To whom much is given, much is expected". Every family should encourage its participants to give to each other and to give back to society in a meaningful way. The world could benefit from more of us sharing our talents and skills. To keep America great we all have to have an attitude of service.

Step 8: *Promote a spiritual life for the family and individual members of the family.* A family that prays together, stays together. God created the family unit as a reflection of love, nurturing, order and expansion of humankind.

Step 9: *Make family time sacred.* Whatever time is set aside daily or weekly for family interactions or gatherings, that time should be protected and kept sacred. Turn off the phones, television and anything that detracts from the quality of the interactions during your "family time." Members of families should not miss graduation, birthday parties, family reunions, wedding, births and deaths.

Step 10: *Make grandparents part of the nuclear family.* Strong families value the participation of grandparents and other extended family members. Grandparents have the time to be good listeners and advisors. In a forest, only those trees with deep roots ever grow tall enough to reach the sun.

# 75

---cv---

# GENTLEMEN ARE NEVER OBESE

*A husband should love his wife as much as*
*Christ loved the Church.*
 Ephesians 5:25

According to the Centers for Disease Control, 61% of adults and 25% of children and adolescents in the United State are overweight. This is primarily due to overeating and to the fact that 40% of us do not engage in leisure physical activities. The dramatic change in overall physique from the past to present can be seen by comparing family photos from the past with photos from today.

Although the media focus has been on the even higher rates of overweight and obesity among African-American women, African-American men also suffer from high rates of excess weight. This excess weight substantially increases the risks of diabetes, stroke, cancer and even arthritis. In fact, obese adults have twice the rate of premature death and disability than the average sized person in the United States. The high rate of obesity among African-American males is unacceptable. African-Americans over seventy years old are not obese. What do you think happened to those who were obese?

Instead of experimenting with fad diets to lose weight and joining health clubs that you never use, doctors currently recommend that you exercise daily and eat a little less. The difference between what an average-sized person and what an obese person consumes is not very much. It turns out that the average obese person eats, or fails to burn up, just 150 excess calories per day. That difference is just about a small bag of potato chips or a can of soda. But it adds up to more that 50,000 extra calories per year that can add five pounds of fat. Over 20 years, the person who is consuming 150 extra calories per day will have added an extra 100 pounds.

Society encourages us to avoid exertion and become sluggards, to take escalators instead of walking up stairs. Older people, who are quite capable of walking, cannot make their way through an airport without repeated offers to push them in a wheelchair. Even when we try to walk somewhere, someone is always offering to drive us. Golfers cannot walk anymore—carts are required.

A gentleman is never obese for many reasons. First of all, gentlemen never eat in fast-food restaurants—how uncivilized! Other than forgiving others for their transgressions, gentlemen generally do not do things quickly. They like to savor the moment, smell the roses and enjoy God's gifts to us. In addition to regular exercise and a prudent diet, men can easily burn up an extra 150 calories per day performing gentlemanly deeds. Actively greeting others, opening car doors, pulling out chairs, putting on coats, carrying packages, grooming ourselves, keeping our cars, shoes and clothes clean and presentable—all of these little courtesies burn calories. Old men are fond of telling young men to always smile at ladies and find opportunities to be helpful and courteous. They delight in rescuing damsels in distress. You may suspect that they did this to win favor with the ladies only to discover that the true motivation is to look sharp and debonair. A sure sign that you are in the presence of a gentleman is if the lady is obese, because a gentleman does everything for his lady.